Update on Surgical Palliative Care

Guest Editor

GEOFFREY P. DUNN, MD, FACS

SURGICAL CLINICS
OF NORTH AMERICA

www.surgical.theclinics.com

Consulting Editor
RONALD F. MARTIN, MD

April 2011 • Volume 91 • Number 2

SAUNDERS an imprint of ELSEVIER, Inc.

W.B. SAUNDERS COMPANY

A Division of Elsevier Inc.

1600 John F. Kennedy Blvd., Suite 1800, Philadelphia, PA 19103-2899

http://www.surgical.theclinics.com

SURGICAL CLINICS OF NORTH AMERICA Volume 91, Number 2
April 2011 ISSN 0039–6109, ISBN-13: 978-1-4557-0508-5

Editor: John Vassallo, j.vassallo@elsevier.com

Developmental Editor: Donald Mumford

Surgical Clinics of North America (ISSN 0039–6109) is published bimonthly by Elsevier Inc., 360 Park Avenue South, New York, NY 10010-1710. Months of publication are February, April, June, August, October, and December. Business and Editorial Offices: 1600 John F. Kennedy Blvd., Suite 1800, Philadelphia, PA 19103-2899. Periodicals postage paid at New York, NY and additional mailing offices. Subscription prices are $311.00 per year for US individuals, $532.00 per year for US institutions, $152.00 per year for US students and residents, $381.00 per year for Canadian individuals, $661.00 per year for Canadian institutions, $429.00 for international individuals, $661.00 per year for international institutions and $210.00 per year for Canadian and foreign students/residents. To receive student/resident rate, orders must be accompanied by name of affiliated institution, date of term, and the *signature* of program/ residency coordinator on institution letterhead. Orders will be billed at individual rate until proof of status is received. Foreign air speed delivery is included in all *Clinics* subscription prices. All prices are subject to change without notice. POSTMASTER: Send address changes to *Surgical Clinics*, Elsevier Health Sciences Division, Subscription Customer Service, 3251 Riverport Lane, Maryland Heights, MO 63043. **Customer Service (orders, claims, online, change of address): Telephone: 1-800-654-2452 (U.S. and Canada); 314-447-8871 (outside U.S. and Canada). Fax: 314-447-8029. E-mail: journalscustomerservice-usa@elsevier.com (for print support); journalsonline support-usa@elsevier.com (for online support).**

Reprints. For copies of 100 or more, of articles in this publication, please contact the Commercial Reprints Department, Elsevier Inc., 360 Park Avenue South, New York, New York 10010-1710. Tel. (212) 633-3812, Fax: (212) 462-1935, e-mail: reprints@elsevier.com.

The Surgical Clinics of North America is also published in Spanish by McGraw-Hill Interamericana Editores S.A., P.O. Box 5-237 06500 Mexico D.F. Mexico; and in Portuguese by Interlivros Edicoes Ltda., Rua Comandante Coelho 1085, CEP 21250, Rio de Janeiro, Brazil; and in Greek by Paschalidis Medical Publications, Athens Greece.

The Surgical Clinics of North America is covered in *MEDLINE/PubMed (Index Medicus), EMBASE/Excerpta Medica, Current Contents/Clinical Medicine, Current Contents/Life Sciences, Science Citation Index,* and *ISI/BIOMED.*

Printed and bound by CPI Group (UK) Ltd, Croydon, CR0 4YY

Transferred to Digital Print 2011

Contributors

CONSULTING EDITOR

RONALD F. MARTIN, MD
Staff Surgeon, Department of Surgery, Marshfield Clinic, Marshfield, Wisconsin; Clinical Associate Professor, University of Wisconsin School of Medicine and Public Health, Madison, Wisconsin; Colonel, Medical Corps, United States Army Reserve

GUEST EDITOR

GEOFFREY P. DUNN, MD, FACS
Department of Surgery and Palliative Care Consultation Service, UPMC Hamot Medical Center, Erie, Pennsylvania

AUTHORS

MICHAEL D. ADOLPH, MD, FACS
Assistant Clinical Professor of Internal Medicine and Surgery, Division of Surgical Oncology, Pain & Palliative Medicine Service, Center for Palliative Care, James Cancer Hospital and Solove Research Institute, The Ohio State University College of Medicine, Columbus, Ohio

EMILY BELLAVANCE, MD
Fellow, Surgical Oncology, Department of Surgery, University of Chicago, Chicago, Illinois

GEOFFREY P. DUNN, MD, FACS
Department of Surgery and Palliative Care Consultation Service, UPMC Hamot Medical Center, Erie, Pennsylvania

CHRISTOPHER P. EVANS, MD, FACS
Professor and Chair, Department of Urology, UC Davis Cancer Center, UC Davis Medical Center, University of California, Davis, Sacramento, California

BETTY FERRELL, PhD, RN, FAAN, MA
Professor and Research Scientist, Department of Population Sciences, Nursing Research and Education, City of Hope, Duarte, California

FRED GRANNIS, MD
Clinical Professor, Department of Surgery; Thoracic Surgeon, Thoracic Cancer Program, City of Hope, Duarte, California

NADER N. HANNA, MD, FACS
Head, Division of Surgical Oncology; Associate Professor of Surgery, University of Maryland School of Medicine, Baltimore, Maryland

ANNIE HARRINGTON, MD
Fellow, Department of Medicine, Division of Pulmonary and Critical Care, Cedars Sinai Medical Center, Los Angeles, California

JOAN L. HUFFMAN, MD, FACS, CWS, FACCWS
Medical Director, Wound Healing Program; Assistant Professor, Division of Acute
Care Surgery, Department of Surgery, University of Florida at Shands Jacksonville,
Jacksonville, Florida

GRETCHEN PURCELL JACKSON, MD, PhD, FACS
Assistant Professor of Surgery, Department of Pediatric Surgery, Vanderbilt Children's
Hospital, Nashville, Tennessee

TIMOTHY KEAY, MD
Professor, Department of Family and Community Medicine, University of Maryland
School of Medicine, Baltimore, Maryland

MARIANNA KOCZYWAS, MD
Associate Professor of Medicine, Division of Medical Oncology and Therapeutics
Research, Thoracic Oncology and Lung Cancer Program, City of Hope, Duarte,
California

FREDERICK J. MEYERS, MD, MACP
Executive Associate Dean, Professor of Internal Medicine and Pathology, Department
of Internal Medicine, UC Davis Cancer Center, UC Davis School of Medicine, University
of California, Davis, Sacramento, California

THOMAS J. MINER, MD
Assistant Professor of Surgery, Associate Program Director, General Surgery; Director
of Surgical Oncology, Department of Surgery, The Alpert Medical School of Brown
University, Rhode Island Hospital, Providence, Rhode Island

ANNE CHARLOTTE MOSENTHAL, MD, FACS
Professor of Surgery, New Jersey Medical School, University of Medicine and Dentistry
of New Jersey, Newark, New Jersey

DAVID W. PAGE, MD, FACS
Professor of Surgery, Clerkship Director in Surgery, Department of Surgery, Tufts
University School of Medicine, Baystate Medical Center, Springfield, Massachusetts

JAY REQUARTH, MD, FACS
Assistant Professor, Section of Vascular and Interventional Radiology, Department
of Radiology, Wake Forest University Baptist Medical Center, Winston Salem,
North Carolina

JULIA SHELTON, MD
Resident Physician, Department of Surgery, Vanderbilt University Medical Center,
Nashville, Tennessee

JOHN L. TARPLEY, MD
Professor of Surgery and Anesthesiology, Program Director, Chief, General Surgery,
Department of Surgery, Vanderbilt University, Veterans Affairs Medical Center Surgical
Service, Veterans Affairs Tennessee Valley Healthcare System, Nashville, Tennessee

MARGARET J. TARPLEY, MLS
Senior Associate in Surgery, Department of Surgery, Vanderbilt University, Nashville,
Tennessee

CHRISTINE C. TOEVS, MD, FACS, FCCM
Roanoke, Virginia

LESLIE STEELE TYRIE, MD
Assistant Professor of Surgery, New Jersey Medical School, University of Medicine and Dentistry of New Jersey, Newark, New Jersey

JENNIFER N. WU, MD
Urology Resident, Department of Urology, UC Davis Cancer Center, UC Davis Medical Center, University of California, Davis, Sacramento, California

Contents

> Palliation has been an essential, if not the primary, activity of surgery during much of its history. However, it has been only during the past decade that the modern principles and practices of palliative care developed in the nonsurgical specialties in the United States and abroad have been introduced to surgical institutions, widely varied practice settings, education, and research.

> The traditional action-oriented surgical personality, although essential in the service of solving emergent operative dilemmas, may serve as a barrier to introspection. Certainly, challenges of the twenty-first century practice environment, including time constraints, also distract from self-reflection. Without engaging in moments of introspection, surgeons risk not only abandoning dying patients in their time of need, but leave the surgeons themselves at risk for burnout and its consequences. The increase in the number of women surgeons, as well as the less heroic image of surgeons performing laparoscopic operations, may reorient traditional extroverted behavior toward a persona of professional grace.

> The spiritual dimensions of surgical palliative care encompass recognition of mortality (physician and patient); knowledge of moral and ethical dilemmas of medical decision making; respect for each individual and for all belief systems; responsibility to remain physically and psychologically present for the patient and family; and knowledge of when chaplains, palliative care professionals, or social workers should be consulted. Certain aspects of surgical palliative care distinguish it from palliative care in other medical disciplines such as the 2 definitions (palliative procedure and palliative care), treating a disproportionate share of patients who suffer unforeseen tragic events, and the surgical system.

Excellence as a surgeon requires not only the technical and intellectual ability to effectively take care of surgical disease but also an ability to respond to the needs and questions of patients. This article provides an overview of the importance of communication skills in optimal surgical palliation and offers suggestions for a multidisciplinary team approach, using the palliative triangle as the ideal model of communication and interpersonal skills. This article also discusses guidelines for advanced surgical decision making and outlines methods to improve communication skills.

The image-guided procedures discussed in this article are used to alleviate pain and suffering of patients with malignancies and/or multiple comorbidities. It is not possible to discuss the entire breadth of image-guided palliative procedures; only a few commonly requested procedures are reviewed: cholecystostomy, biliary decompression, enteral feeding and decompression tubes, chemical neurolysis (for pain control), cementoplasty, tunneled drainage catheters, transjugular intrahepatic portasystemic shunt pleurodesis, tube thoracostomy, thermal and chemical tumor ablation, transcatheter arterial chemoembolization, and selective internal radiation therapy. A decision tree is given with each procedure/disease. This review provides referring surgeons a framework for end-of-life treatment and palliation discussions.

Advancements in the surgical and medical treatment of lung cancer have resulted in more favorable short-term survival outcomes. After initial treatment, lung cancer requires continued surveillance and follow-up for long-term side effects and possible recurrence. The integration of quality palliative care into routine clinical care of patients with lung cancer after surgical intervention is essential in preserving function and optimizing quality of life through survivorship. An interdisciplinary palliative care model can effectively link patients to the appropriate supportive care services in a timely fashion. This article describes the role of palliative care for patients with lung cancer.

Pediatric surgeons can play an important role in offering procedures that may improve the quality of life for terminally ill children. As with all palliative interventions, surgical therapies should be evaluated in the context of explicitly defined treatment goals while weighing the risks and benefits of procedures in the context of a shortened life span. It is essential that pediatric surgeons become active members in the multidisciplinary team that provides palliative care.

> Urological malignancies, especially prostate cancer, are relatively common, but patients may live many years before eventually dying of the disease. Caring for these patients is an important role for urologists, although medical training often does not adequately prepare urologists for the palliative care of patients with advanced malignancies. Palliative care is no longer equated with end-of-life care, but rather integrated throughout illness, even when cure is impossible. This article focuses on the various palliative treatments available for the 3 most common urological malignancies: prostate, bladder, and renal cancers.

> Palliative care in itself has many challenges; these challenges are compounded exponentially when placed in the setting of a mass casualty event, such as the 2010 Haiti earthquake. Haiti itself was an austere environment with very little infrastructure before the disaster. US surgeons, intensivists, and nurses worked hand in hand with other international providers and Haitian volunteers to provide the best care for the many. Improvisation and teamwork as well as respect for the Haitian caregivers were crucial to their successes. Sisyphean trials lie ahead. Haiti and its people must not be forgotten.

THE CLINICS ARE NOW AVAILABLE ONLINE!

Access your subscription at:
www.theclinics.com

Foreword

Update on Surgical Palliative Care

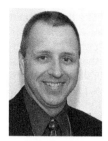

Ronald F. Martin, MD
Consulting Editor

The irony of writing this foreword for an issue on *Surgical Palliative Care* from a hostile fire zone is not lost on me given the antithetical nature of hostility to palliation. The very essence of palliation is, in my opinion, the willingness to do those things that ease the suffering of people first and foremost whether those acts contribute to eliminating the underlying problem or not. In many respects, palliative efforts reflect the nature of true human caring. At its core, thinking about our discipline in a "palliative" way forces us to differentiate between what we can do and what we should do.

The forces at play near the end of life, no matter how slowly or suddenly that approaches a patient, are usually complex but similar. When we are confronted with these unsolvable problems, we progress from shock and denial to acceptance and progression, for the most part, whether we wish to or not. Clearly, end-of-life issues most greatly affect the patient, whom we are directly (and I would argue most) responsible to serve. That stated, the impact on the families and loved ones, the areas where decision-making involves legal matters, and the impact and involvement of the medical team cannot and should not be ignored. Once a patient enters the health care system, the interaction itself develops a life of its own and a story of its own. And like other stories, some will be shorter or longer than others, but all will have a beginning, a middle, and an end.

My personal observation has been that there is tremendous variety to how these "stories of medical involvement" are written depending upon the physician who is responsible for the patient's care. I suppose that is to be expected to some degree. There are the full-speed-ahead-no-matter-what stylists and there are the nihilists and all manner of in-between stylists. Perhaps there is a role for all of these approaches, but I would argue that the story line should be more dependent on the patient's desires than the desires of the physician.

In this era of complicated and fractionated care, especially when a patient may frequently move back and forth between the inpatient and outpatient environment,

Surg Clin N Am 91 (2011) xiii–xv
doi:10.1016/j.suc.2011.01.007
0039-6109/11/$ – see front matter © 2011 Elsevier Inc. All rights reserved.

maintaining the overall goal of care appears to be more fragile than ever. The number of "handoffs" and potential areas for breakdown in communication exacerbate the problems in continuing a sound plan. Also, the development of relationships seems to be a continuous reinvention, frequently within a single hospital admission for some patients. Patients, families, nurses, physicians, and other members of the team all become frustrated when goals and objectives become or remain unclear, which only serves to make difficult situations more difficult.

Another observation that has struck me is that physicians don't like to talk about death, in particular, physicians from the United States of America. I count myself among them—I don't care for it too much. The old adage tells of two certainties: death and taxes. I hear a great deal of chatter from my colleagues about the latter and not a whole lot about the former. And perhaps it is due to our cultural reluctance to address death, because either we fear it, consider it a failure, or we are just uncomfortable with how to discuss it, that we sometimes fail to develop an informed understanding of what our patients want for options and limits of care instead of what we think they should have.

As with many things we must do that are uncomfortable or difficult, they generally get easier with having some basic tools with which to work and some opportunity to practice. The more one takes the time to explore these difficult topics with patients and their families, the easier it becomes to do so; although I doubt it ever becomes easy. Dr Dunn, who among other things I consider a truly decent man and a valued friend, has really done our surgical community a lifetime of service in tackling these challenging topics. His work for the American College of Surgeons should be reviewed and considered by anyone who cares for patients. He and his colleagues have assembled a collection of articles that will dispel some of the myths about surgeons as palliators and will give the reader a set of tools to more effectively address some of these challenging issues.

On a slightly tangential note, perspective is an interesting thing. As alluded to, I am currently away from my usual environment. Here in the mountains of Afghanistan, one has a real opportunity to see what differences there are in expectations. There is something in the military we call Medical Rules of Eligibility or MROE. The MROE are what we use to basically determine who gets what. The MROE exist because the chain of command in our military has accepted that we cannot be all things at all times for everyone and, therefore, there will be a code that delineates how we will, for want of a better word, ration care. I shall not presume to tell anybody what to think of such a process or how to feel about it. These rules allow us to make decisions based on some very stark realities that different groups and different countries or organizations quite simply have different levels of access to resources and differing expectations about what their collective group will or can spare on behalf of an individual. For US military personnel, the resources available (including evacuation, of course) are the totality of efforts that we as a country can bring to bear. For the local citizens, the options are far more varied. In the acute setting, especially when it comes to "life, limb, or eyesight," the differences are small. Despite what some may write or say, there is a very good chance that if someone makes it to a US facility with any injury of significance they will receive initial care—we have rules about that. The differences really begin to become apparent when one is past that initial phase of care and will be moving on to the host country's regular resources. Expenditures that we would consider routine in the United States are simply inconceivable in other environments.

Despite these variations in allocations, the local people whom we have had the opportunity to care for have been uniformly grateful for anything we have done for them. Even though we have done far less in some cases than we might have been able to do at "home," we have exceeded their expectations here. And in all circumstances, there has been a deep appreciation that we cared enough to even try.

At the end of the day the business of patient care is about caring for the patient. It is not necessarily about doing things *to* them as much as making sure that we do things *for* them. With all the talk of patient-centered medical home models and accountable care organizations as well as other efforts we will undertake that will do more to alter reimbursement in some situations than patient outcomes, we would do well to remember that none of us gets out of here alive. Perhaps focusing on the quality of the end game is as important in some regards as focusing on how to stave it off.

Ronald F. Martin, MD
COL, USAR, MC
Chief of Surgery
1982 Forward Surgical Team (forward)
FOB Shank, Afghanistan

Department of Surgery
Marshfield Clinic
1000 North Oak Avenue
Marshfield, WI 54449, USA

E-mail address:
martin.ronald@marchfieldclinic.org

Preface

Update on Surgical Palliative Care

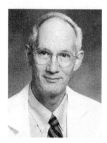

Geoffrey P. Dunn, MD
Guest Editor

Since the publication of the last *Surgical Clinics of North America* volume on surgical palliative care in April 2005, palliative care principles and practices have been increasingly recognized and integrated into the practice and institutions of surgery. During this time, the more general field of palliative care has established itself as a medical subspecialty and has created a high educational standard for itself through the establishment of over sixty fellowship programs and numerous other educational initiatives. Basic research is rapidly proliferating, although still lags in funding appropriate for the potential benefits. Hospital palliative care programs are rapidly proliferating while the National Quality Forum has identified quality indicators and best practices. Despite the recent political setback of the "death panel" characterization of federal funding for the most innocent of all medical interventions, the patient/doctor discussion about end-of-life treatment preferences, favorable public perception of palliative care is increasing, in part, due to the popular writings of surgeons Pauline Chen and Atul Gawande. Palliative care has become a timely lens through which the socioeconomic and spiritual bankruptcy of the current health care system and our prevailing expectations of the health care system are starkly visible especially when it is focused on the hospital care of patients with advanced and critical illness.

This volume demonstrates the diversity of application of the fundamental principles of palliative care to varied surgical specialties and settings. The articles have been selected to provide more depth to the philosophical and spiritual basis for this patient-centered approach, while presenting widely varying scenarios for application of its principles. After an introductory summary of changes in the field of palliative care relevant to surgeons, two articles follow that encourage surgeons to look inward as a prerequisite for effective presence to our patients when the goal is the mitigation of suffering and the reaffirmation of hope. This prerequisite is not asked for lightly, recognizing that surgeons have traditionally prided themselves more for their capacity to act

Surg Clin N Am 91 (2011) xvii–xviii
doi:10.1016/j.suc.2011.01.005
0039-6109/11/$ – see front matter © 2011 Elsevier Inc. All rights reserved.

decisively than to indulge in introspection. Introspection is not, however, indulgent if it is the basis for effective counsel and action as it so often is in critical, life-limiting, or terminal illness. Dr Adolph's article introduces the reader to the daily world of the palliative care consultant, highlighting the importance of the interdisciplinary process.

Several venues of surgical palliative care and their associated issues are then exhibited: the status of palliative care in the critical care setting is summarized by Dr Toevs, while Dr Mosenthal and coworkers explore the underappreciated issue of bereavement associated with critical illness. Dr Hanna's article demonstrates how congruous and necessary palliative considerations are for all oncologic care, not just those in the last phases of illness. Dr Miner, already well known for his pioneering work in defining palliative surgery and its outcomes, shares his insights into framing the palliative surgery discussion, which could be considered an operation itself. Dr Requarth, a surgeon and an interventional radiologist, catalogues the extensive repertoire of interventions available as alternatives to open and laparoscopic surgical procedures. Dr Ferrell and colleagues, pioneers in advocating palliative care for surgical patients, shares their institution's experience with palliative support of patients with lung cancer, which recent evidence suggests, that in addition to standard oncologic therapy, cannot only improve quality of life, but also survival outcomes. Dr Jackson and colleagues and Dr Wu and coworkers then review palliative aspects of two surgical subspecialties, pediatric surgery and urology, for which there has been little previous guidance. The volume concludes with Dr Huffman's riveting account of her experience last year in earthquake-devastated Haiti, which demonstrates the very essence of surgical palliative care—an intuitive response to the mitigation of suffering and the restoration of hope using the insights and skills we are privileged to have and share as surgeons.

What has changed since 2005 has been the increased recognition that palliative care restores the hope to live in peace, not piecemeal, for all seriously ill patients, and not just those at the end of life. The surgical world has too many seriously ill people in its care and too much to offer the seriously ill with all diagnoses to not assume a leadership role for the continued growth and development of palliative care. Recent developments in the field of surgery such as shown in this volume give reason for optimism that this will occur.

Geoffrey P. Dunn, MD
Department of Surgery and
Palliative Care Consultation Service
UPMC Hamot Medical Center
2050 South Shore Drive
Erie, PA 16505, USA

E-mail address:
gpdunn1@earthlink.net

Dedication

This volume is dedicated to Jack M. Zimmerman, MD, FACS, a pioneer of hospice and palliative care in the United States. Dr Zimmerman, while Chief of Surgery at Church Home and Hospital and consulting at Johns Hopkins Hospital in the 1970s, was instrumental in establishing one of the first hospice programs in the United States at the Church Home and Hospital. He was a seminal contributor to the surgical literature on this topic and wrote one of the earliest clinical textbooks on hospice care, *Hospice: Complete Care of the Terminally Ill*, in 1981. His instinctive sense of the importance of palliative care in surgical and medical practice and his success in its implementation stand as a model for all surgeons to emulate.

Geoffrey P. Dunn

Surg Clin N Am 91 (2011) xix
doi:10.1016/j.suc.2011.01.006
0039-6109/11/$ – see front matter © 2011 Elsevier Inc. All rights reserved.

Surgical Palliative Care: Recent Trends and Developments

Geoffrey P. Dunn, MD

KEYWORDS

• Palliative care • Surgical palliative care • Palliative surgery
• Symptom management • End-of-life care

VIGNETTES: THEN AND NOW
1985

A 55-year-old woman with a history of stage III ovarian carcinoma, 1 year after total abdominal hysterectomy, bilateral salpingo-oophorectomy and omentectomy, and several cycles of cisplatin-based chemotherapy, presents at a 350-bed regional medical center with increasing abdominal pain and distention, nausea, and vomiting. She was told she was stable at her last outpatient oncology evaluation 2 months previously when she was complaining of abdominal pain, numbness in her feet, and loss of appetite. She is receiving no regular medications except propoxyphene with acetaminophen (Darvocet) as needed for abdominal pain. On physical examination she is pale and cachectic. She has diminished breath sounds with dullness to percussion at each lung base, more so on the right. Her abdomen is distended with a remote midline incision.

Bowel sounds are high pitched. She has shifting dullness to percussion and multiple palpable abdominal masses. She has no guarding. Plain abdominal radiographs are consistent with a small-bowel obstruction. Bilateral moderate-sized pleural effusions are noted on the chest radiograph. The surgeon tells her he thinks she has a bowel obstruction from her cancer and he would like to avoid operating if at all possible. A nasogastric (NG) tube is inserted and placed to continuous suction. She is not given opioid analgesia because of the surgeon's fear of masking peritoneal signs. After 5 days of nonoperative therapy the patient is advised that her condition mandates surgery because of persistent obstruction and fears of potential gangrenous bowel. She signs an operative consent for exploratory laparotomy, possible bowel resection, removal of tumor, possible formation of ostomy, and insertion of central venous catheter. Potential complications listed include failure to remove the entire tumor,

The author has nothing to disclose.
Department of Surgery, Palliative Care Consultation Service, UPMC Hamot Medical Center, Erie, PA, USA
E-mail address: gpdunn1@earthlink.net

Surg Clin N Am 91 (2011) 277–292
doi:10.1016/j.suc.2011.01.002
0039-6109/11/$ – see front matter © 2011 Elsevier Inc. All rights reserved.

surgical.theclinics.com

reobstruction, bleeding, bowel injury, wound hernia, fistula formation, and pneumothorax. The patient confides to her nurse that she is worried the surgeon, "will not be able to remove all of the tumor." The patient proceeds to an exploratory laparotomy by an experienced general surgeon assisted by a third-year surgical resident. While at the scrub sink, the surgeon tells the resident, "This will probably be an exercise in futility. I feel like an executioner. At least this way, she might not live the rest of her life with an NG tube stuck down her nose." After making a generous midline incision, a large amount of ascites and multiple points of small-bowel obstruction secondary to bulky tumor are noted. Additionally, extensive studding of all peritoneal surfaces with tumor is noted. A gastrostomy for drainage is placed and subclavian venous access is established for administration of total parenteral nutrition. The surgeon discloses the findings to the patient's husband in a busy waiting room. "Unfortunately, there was nothing we could do but palliate her with a gastrostomy tube. We will see what the oncologists can recommend and give her intravenous nutrition so she will not starve." The following day, the same findings are disclosed to the patient in the same fashion as disclosed to her husband by the surgeon during morning rounds. The patient asks, "What happens next?" to which the surgeon responds, "It's in God's hands at this point." The patient's postoperative analgesia orders specify meperidine 25 to 50 mg intramuscularly (IM) every 3 hours as needed and hydroxyzine 25 mg IM every 3 hours as needed. The consulting oncologist tells the patient he would like to defer chemotherapy until the patient "becomes stronger." A close friend of the patient privately asks the surgeon, "what he knows about hospice," to which he scornfully responds, "What are they going to do for her, kill her with morphine?" On the fourth postoperative day, bilious drainage begins draining from the midline incision at the site of an external retention suture, which necessitates placement of an ostomy drainage bag. Two days later, the patient becomes lethargic, hypotensive, and anuric and is transferred to the surgical intensive care unit (SICU). Because of the hypotension, her nurse withholds her pain medication but exhorts her to "not give up." Because of ongoing hypotension and hypoxemia, an arterial line and Swan-Ganz catheter are inserted, vasopressor support is initiated, and the patient is intubated for ventilator support. She receives multiple infusions of albumin and frequent boluses of crystalloid. A right-sided thoracostomy tube is placed because of an increasingly large pleural effusion. After 2 days, the patient becomes increasingly obtunded and hypotensive, and then develops ventricular ectopy, which is followed by ventricular fibrillation. She is defibrillated but is unable to resume a cardiac rhythm and is pronounced dead by the ICU resident. The family is notified by telephone and asked to come to the hospital for her personal effects. One week later her case is presented at the surgical department's mortality and morbidity rounds because of her postoperative complication and death. The consensus of the surgeons present is "What else could you [the surgeon] do?"

2010

A 55-year-old woman with a history of stage III ovarian carcinoma, 3 years status after total abdominal hysterectomy, bilateral salpingo-oophorectomy and omentectomy, and subsequent carboplatin, paclitaxel, and topotecan chemotherapy presents at a 350-bed regional medical center with increasing abdominal distention, abdominal pain, nausea, and vomiting. Further questioning reveals she has dyspnea and profound weakness. She is an active member of an ovarian cancer support group facilitated by a health care professional. A palliative care team at the outpatient cancer treatment center actively follows her for management of her cancer-related pain and chemotherapy-induced neuropathic pain. She is receiving 160 mg extended-release morphine daily, with 20 mg immediate-release morphine every 2 hours as needed for breakthrough pain and gabapentin 600 mg daily for her neuropathic pain. Additionally, she is taking megestrol acetate 600 mg daily for appetite stimulation and mirtazapine15 mg daily for depression and sleeplessness.

At the time of her admission, her surgeon assesses her pain during which she reports generalized abdominal pain with an intensity of 8 to 9 out of 10 with pain spikes "above 10." Her pain was well controlled 1 week previously. On physical examination she is pale and cachectic. She has diminished breath sounds with dullness to percussion at each lung base, more so on the right. Her abdomen is distended with a remote midline incision.

Bowel sounds are high pitched. She has shifting dullness to percussion and multiple palpable abdominal masses. She has no guarding. The surgeon explains to the patient that he would like to make her more comfortable before initiating any diagnostics or conversation to which she promptly agrees. He orders morphine 20 mg intravenously (IV) every 4 hours with 10 mg IV every 2 hours as needed for breakthrough pain. Following this, a nasogastric tube is inserted and two liters of bilious fluid is drained.

The surgeon explains to her that he will now order a CT scan of the abdomen and pelvis with contrast to determine the site of obstruction, its probable cause, and extent of her disease. He asks her to invite others of her choosing to be present later when he discusses the results in her room. He states that he is concerned that among the possible reasons for her clinical presentation is progressing disease, in which case several important decisions will have to be made. The patient indicates she will have her husband present. CT of the abdomen and pelvis shows evidence of small-bowel obstruction, a small amount of ascites, and disseminated bulky disease. She also is noted to have a large right pleural effusion. Laboratory results include prealbumin (7 mg/dL), hematocrit (23%), and CA 125 (7000 U/mL). The surgeon asks the patient's nurse to accompany him during his meeting with the patient and her husband. He turns off his beeper, introduces himself to the patient's husband and sits down in a chair next to the patient. After he determines that her pain is now well controlled ("2 out of 10, much better"), the surgeon asks them what they already know about her illness and if they are willing to hear any new important information. Both indicate their willingness to proceed with the discussion. The patient says, "I know it isn't looking good, my oncologist said we have about run out of options. My CA 125 has been going up but I am hoping it's the chemo that has been making me so weak and sick. My support group has been telling me to seek another opinion. I don't want to give up for my family's sake," looking pleadingly at her husband, "but I don't think I can do this anymore." The surgeon acknowledges how difficult this must be with her physical discomfort and her concerns for her family. The husband speaks up and says, tearfully, "I just don't want her to suffer." The surgeon acknowledges that he can see that this is his wish. He then tells them that the scan and blood tests have confirmed their fears, that the cancer has significantly progressed and has now caused a bowel blockage. He tells them there is also a large amount of fluid in the right chest cavity. The surgeon remains silent as she reacts to the news with a knowing downward look nodding her head and crying softly. He offers her a tissue and states, "I can see this has come as a sad disappointment to you," turning to the husband, "and you." After a long period of silence she states, "what next?" The husband asks if surgery can relieve her blockage. The surgeon says, "Let's go back to what you said about your wish that she not suffer and use that as the standard by which we decide what to do and what not do. Surgery is theoretically possible, although I am not recommending it for several reasons. She has some of the features that predict poor survival and quality-of-life outcomes from surgery in this situation: the fluid in her abdomen; the multiple bulky masses; and most importantly, the failure of multiple chemotherapy regimens to control the disease. Additionally, she has poor nutritional status, and, as she has said she is tired, in the sense that her reserves are exhausted. Even if surgery relieved her blockage, it will not restore her strength or appetite." The patient's husband looks bewildered and states, "What do you do if you don't operate and she can't eat?" The surgeon responds, "Let me break this down into several answers because there are several forms of discomfort or suffering her illness can cause. We can relieve her of the symptoms of bowel obstruction and the fluid in her abdomen and chest cavities using a combination of medications and procedures less invasive than an open operation. While this is getting underway, we will work on preparing for your ongoing support after she is out of the hospital. Your question about eating is more of a challenge because we equate eating with health and survival and food is such a central part of the way we relate to others. The lack of appetite and the ability for the body to turn nutrients into beneficial protein is a part of her illness. It's not lack of food that is making her ill, it's her illness that is now making the benefit of food impossible, which is not starving in the usual sense of the word. The word *starving* implies that the restoration of lacking nutrients would reverse the condition. That is, unfortunately, not the case here." The surgeon continues, looking at the husband, "You may be less distressed to know that she is probably indifferent to food and would be relieved to not have it be the focus at this point." The patient nods affirmatively. The surgeon concludes by explaining the regimen of medications he will use to give her relief from her bowel obstruction, explaining that she may have an occasional emesis but that is generally acceptable to patients if their nausea and pain are controlled. He then tells her he will be in again later to see if she is getting relief and to answer further questions. In addition to the morphine she is receiving, he orders octreotide 250 µg subcutaneously every 12 hours and prochlorperazine 10 mg IV every 6 hours, and then removes her nasogastric tube. When he returns several hours later she is comfortable. She tells the surgeon, "I want to go home." The surgeon confirms with them that they have accepted his recommendation not to have surgery and instead focus on keeping her comfortable and expediting her return home. He states that he is confident that she can be kept comfortable in her home setting with the proper support. She then asks him, "How long can this go?" The surgeon asks the patient and her husband if they are ready to discuss prognosis at this time, to which they both respond definitely yes. The surgeon says, "When we give estimates, we are giving averages of all patients with similar problems, not necessarily what will happen to you. Our best way of making an estimate is the change in the person's functional status, in other words, what you are able to do during a day. If you are bedbound and with a known progressive, life-limiting illness such as yours and requiring total care, survival is measured in weeks or less." Silence follows. The surgeon tells them, "I can see how sad this is making you." The patient says, "Actually, that is what I figured. When can I go?" The surgeon responds by telling them she could leave as soon as her home is ready and her symptoms are reliably controlled. He tells them that the best support available to fulfill her wish to be home and keep her symptoms controlled would be a hospice program. The surgeon tells them it would be prudent to clarify at this time her future preferences for interventions, such as cardiopulmonary resuscitation, ventilator support, intravenous hydration, and artificial nutrition. The patient says she is no longer interested in these interventions, to which the surgeon responds that he supports her preferences because of the marginal benefit these interventions would bestow during this phase of her illness. He asks them if they think they have the spiritual support they would want at this time, to which they respond they have already met with their pastor earlier in the day. Although her medication is controlling her symptoms well, the patient elects an endoscopic percutaneous gastrostomy (PEG) insertion for drainage. Additionally, the right pleural effusion is drained under CT guidance. Arrangements with a home hospice agency are subsequently made and she returns home the day following PEG placement. Her symptoms remain controlled at home and she is even able to eat small amounts of low-residue food. She succumbs 10 days later, peacefully, surrounded by her family. Several days later, during calling hours before her funeral, the patient's husband gives the surgeon a long silent hug when the surgeon greets him. He says to the surgeon, "You could not have done more for me and my wife."

Palliation has been an essential, if not the primary, activity of surgery during much of its history. However, it has been only during the past decade that the modern principles and practices of palliative care, which were developed in nonsurgical specialties in the United States and abroad, have been introduced to surgical institutions, widely varied practice settings, education, and research.

The experience and success of the hospice movement in the United States and abroad undoubtedly has facilitated the acceptance and development of the field of palliative medicine, although not without some resistance from all medical specialties and the public because of hospice's association with the dying process and the persistence of a death-denying popular and medical culture. The conceptual and psychological challenge for surgeons is the assimilation of principles (patient/family unit as the unit of care, relief of suffering, spiritual growth) first learned from hospice care, which were subsequently adapted to the much larger population of patients with advanced, but not necessarily terminal, illness. This reframing of the goal of care requires a shift from the biophysical (disease-focused) model to a model centered upon suffering or existential considerations independent of the treatment's impact upon the disease processes.

Palliative care is interdisciplinary care that aims to relieve suffering and improve quality of life for patients and their families in the context of serious illness. It is offered simultaneously with all other appropriate medical treatment and its indication is not limited to situations associated with a poor prognosis for survival. Palliative care strives to achieve more than symptom control, but it should not be confused with noncurative treatment. Palliative care is not the opposite of curative treatment. Noncurative treatment is the opposite of curative treatment. *Surgical* palliative care is the treatment of suffering and the promotion of quality of life for patients who are seriously or terminally ill under surgical care (**Table 1**).[1]

The previous strongly contrasting vignettes, taken directly from the author's clinical experience, demonstrate the impact of the growing field of palliative care on surgical practice. Many of the interventions; communication approaches; and the scientific, ethical, and legal underpinnings for the care demonstrated in the second vignette were not available or well developed as recently as the 1990s, and in many hospitals, not even in the last decade. What has changed for surgeons in the interim is their growing capacity to respond to the complexity and potential of patients' experience of serious illness rather than narrowing the scope of the patient encounter by conceptualizing it as management of stage IV disease. Using the operation as the ultimate metaphor for surgeons, the physical operation used to manage a terminal situation in 1985 has evolved into a more expanded concept of the operation, an interdisciplinary exercise that restores comfort, dignity, and hope. This evolution could not have occurred, however, without a concurrent shift in the public and the courts' perception of death.

PALLIATIVE MEDICINE: ITS RECOGNITION AND LEGITIMIZATION IN MEDICAL PRACTICE

Palliative medicine was first recognized as a medical specialty in the United Kingdom where it evolved from the modern hospice movement that also began there during the

Table 1 Palliative care definitions	
Palliative care	Medical care provided by an interdisciplinary team, including the professions of medicine, nursing, social work, chaplaincy, counseling, nursing assistant, and other health care professions, focused on the relief of suffering and support for the best possible quality of life for patients facing serious life-threatening illness and their families. It aims to identify and address the physical, psychological, spiritual, and practical burdens of illness.[45]
Palliative medicine	Palliative medicine is the study and management of patients with active, progressive, and far-advanced disease, for which the prognosis is limited and the focus of care is the quality of life.[46]
Surgical palliative care	*Surgical* palliative care is the treatment of suffering and the promotion of quality of life for patients who are seriously or terminally ill under surgical care.[1]
Palliative surgery	A surgical procedure used with the primary intention of improving quality of life or relieving symptoms caused by advanced disease. Its effectiveness is judged by the presence and durability of patient-acknowledged symptom resolution.
Hospice	*Hospice* is variably used to describe a (1) philosophy of care, (2) a place of care, or (3) an insurance benefit, such as the Medicare Hospice Benefit. Hospice describes supportive care for patients and their families during the patients' final phase of life-limiting illness. The traditional goal of hospice care is to enable patients to be comfortable and free of pain, so that they live each day as contentedly as possible.

1960s and 1970s. It was recognized in Great Britain as a medical subspecialty as early as 1987. Balfour Mount, a urologic oncologist, established the world's first acute care hospital in-patient palliative care service at the Royal Victoria Hospital in Montreal in 1974. His prescient work anticipated the need for these services in an acute care (and surgical) environment that is only now being validated by outcomes studies. He coined the term, *palliative care*.[2] About that time, the first hospice program was established in the United States and the hospice movement was well established here before the field organized and differentiated itself sufficiently to evolve into a medical subspecialty.

The organizational beginnings of the specialty of hospice and palliative medicine in the United States occurred in 1988 when 250 physicians formed the Academy of Hospice Physicians. By the end of 1996, the organization had grown, changed its name to the American Academy of Hospice and Palliative Medicine (AAHPM), and sponsored the American Board of Hospice and Palliative Medicine (ABHPM). The ABHPM independently gave its first certifying examination in November 1996. As of 2006, The American Board of Medical Specialties (ABMS) and its affiliated sponsoring boards have superseded the certification process previously sponsored by ABHPM.

In 2006, the AAHPM and the American Board of Hospice and Palliative Medicine jointly succeeded in achieving recognition of the subspecialty of hospice and palliative medicine within the ABMS and the Accreditation Council for Graduate Medical

Education (ACGME). Ten ABMS boards, including the American Board of Surgery, were subsequently authorized to confer ABMS certification for hospice and palliative medicine. ABMS reported a total of 1271 physicians who successfully received subspecialty certification in hospice and palliative medicine from one of the 10 cosponsoring boards following the first examination in 2008.[3] Following the recognition of hospice and palliative medicine by ABMS and ACGME, The Center for Medicare and Medicaid Services followed suit in 2008. During the past several years, the number of fellowships in palliative medicine has increased (as of January 2010) to a total of 74 active programs offering 181 fellowship positions, including 27 research slots. ACGME has accredited 73 of these programs. After October 2012, only those who have completed an ACGME-accredited fellowship in palliative medicine will be able to sit for the ABMS certification examination. The small number of participants emerging from palliative medicine fellowships who could be certified and those currently certified will not be adequate to respond to the needs of the nation's increasing numbers of hospice and palliative care programs. The looming certified palliative specialist shortfall should prompt practicing physicians and surgeons who are not certified in palliative medicine to familiarize themselves with the basic principles and practices of palliative care as they apply to their respective disciplines. Because the number of surgeons who will pursue fellowships in hospice and palliative medicine will be small, surgeons will have to rely on nonsurgeon palliative medicine specialists for guidance in research design, quality improvement initiatives, and promotion of palliative care.

Other developments critical for the alignment of palliative care with mainstream medicine and positioning it for further introduction into the health care continuum has been the issuance of guidelines and preferred practices. In 2001, with foundation funding, The National Consensus Project for Quality Palliative Care initiative was launched with members representing the leading 5 hospice and palliative care organizations in the United States. Consensus guidelines were subsequently issued in 2004.[4] Using these guidelines as a foundation (**Box 1**), The National Quality Forum established its *National Framework and Preferred Practices for Palliative and Hospice Care.*[5]

The palliative care movement has been shaped and accelerated by changing demographics, failures of the current health care system, the strengthening of individual's autonomy in end-of-life matters in judicial opinion during the past 3 decades, and the favorable popular impact of the hospice movement. In addition, considerable investment by private philanthropic organizations, including the Robert Wood Johnson Foundation[6] and The Open Society Institute[7] founded by George Soros, provided the support necessary to develop the infrastructure and maintain the momentum of the field following the earlier success of hospice whose launching was also greatly benefited by private philanthropic funding before the passage of the Medicare Hospice Benefit in 1983. The success in leveraging millions of dollars of federal support by the private sector for the dying stands out as an instructive and encouraging example for future initiatives related to revision of the health care system. Formerly rapidly fatal diseases, such as cancer, cardiovascular disease, and HIV, have become chronic, life-limiting illnesses. This development has contributed to the expansion of the elderly population that has contributed to the dramatically increasing and unsustainable per capita expenditures[8] for costly new technologies and drugs. An unforeseen consequence of technological success has been the fragmentation of medical care from the subspecialization that has accompanied these advances. This fragmentation is undermining primary care that has historically been the specialty of knowing the individual in their medical and social context. The erosion

---

Box 1
National Quality Forum's 8 domains of quality palliative and hospice care

1. Structures and processes of care

2. Physical aspects of care

3. Psychological and psychiatric aspects of care

4. Social aspects of care

5. Spiritual, religious, and existential aspects of care

6. Cultural aspects of care

7. Care of patients who are imminently dying

8. Ethical and legal aspects of care

From National Quality Forum. A national framework and preferred practices for palliative and hospice care quality. A consensus report. Washington, DC: National Quality Forum; 2006. Available at: http://www.qualityforum.org/Publications/2006/12/A_National_Framework_and_Preferred_Practices_for_Palliative_and_Hospice_Care_Quality.aspx. Accessed January 14, 2011; with permission.

---

of primary care has too often left no effective physician advocate for patients in situations where vision and guidance far beyond the repertoire of surgery and medications are needed. Finally, there has been increased recognition of family caregivers and their unmet practical, social, and psychological needs.[9] Because of its patient/family focus; its emphasis on quality of life; and its recognition of the importance of social, psychological, and spiritual needs, palliative care appears suited to respond to many of these needs and to correct some of the failings of the current health care system.

Given these developments, palliative care programs have not surprisingly proliferated in the United States during the past decade. As of 2008, 53% of hospitals with more than 50 beds in the United States had a palliative care program.[10] Most of these are in-hospital programs, although nursing homes, outpatient treatment centers, and Veterans Affairs hospitals are offering these services. Two initiatives, the Center to Advance Palliative Care[11] and the Veterans Affairs Hospice and Palliative Care Initiative,[12] have greatly facilitated the introduction of palliative care into the in-hospital setting. As the concept has expanded across the spectrum of health care settings, it has also penetrated more than a dozen medical subspecialties in varying degrees whether through sponsorship of the American Board of Internal Medicine subspecialty certification in hospice and palliative medicine or attention to palliative care in position papers, specialty meetings, and journals.

One of the most notable trends, particularly relevant to surgeons, has been the acceptance of palliative care in the critical care setting (see article by Christine C. Toevs elsewhere in this issue for further exploration of this topic). This acceptance might have been inconceivable to many a decade ago, although certainly not surprising given the similarity of illness severity of patients served in the ICU and patients considered suitable for palliative care elsewhere. Palliative care and critical care have 4 fundamental similarities: (1) Both have a strong tradition of team-based care. (2) Both identify patients and families as a unit, which has been a longstanding precept of palliative care for philosophic reasons related to social and psychologic support of patients, while the patient/family is establishing itself as a treatment unit in critical care medicine because of the practical and legal necessity to turn to surrogates for direction and future care planning. Wall and colleagues[13] noted that family satisfaction in the ICU setting was higher for patients that died in the ICU than for families of survivors. They speculate that the increased attention by staff to families of non-survivors was the reason. (3) Both palliative care and critical care recognize that symptom control is mandatory for improvement of function even if only for the function of hope. (4) Both recognize and emphasize the role of communication. Good communication skills, a prerequisite for all palliative care, have recently received closer attention in critical care.[14] There is a high incidence (~30%) of posttraumatic stress disorder (PTSD) among families of ICU survivors, and evidence that the risk of PTSD can be ameliorated by communication with family before patients die or leave the ICU alive.[15] Two models of palliative care have been proposed for the ICU setting: the consultative model uses palliative care consultants to work with ICU staff to guide patients/families identified as not likely to survive the hospitalization and the integrative model seeks to incorporate palliative care principles and interventions in the daily practice of the intensive care unit team for all patients and families facing critical illness.[16]

For surgeons, burn care is the most obvious model for what critical palliative care should look like. It is an outstanding model for palliative care because the care of patients is not based on prognosis but their need for comfort while attempting to preserve or improve function. There is arguably no experience for patients who are critically ill that compares with a major burn for registering extremely high levels of distress in all dimensions of perception (physical, psychological, socioeconomic, and spiritual). Burns are truly a transformative experience for all involved for that reason and for some an end-of-life article. Until recently, burn care was the only surgical care where narcotics were routinely liberally and appropriately employed if for no other reason to make patients manageable and functional as they would be for patients receiving palliative care. This principle was established early on in the hospice movement: the relief of pain is a major prerequisite to the restoration of hope.

Over the past decade, increasing evidence has documented the social, psychological, economic, and even survival benefits for patients in the hospital and outpatient setting resulting from palliative care consultation and interventions. Palliative care has been shown to be patient-centered, beneficial, safe and not associated with earlier death, and more efficient in the use of health care resources and cost. Hospice care received substantially higher satisfaction ratings by families of decedents when compared with standard home health care, hospital care, and nursing home care.[9] Given this finding, it is not surprising that several studies have shown that palliative care improves pain and nonpain symptom control and family satisfaction with care in the public and Veterans' hospital settings.[17–20]

For years, palliative care professionals have suspected that palliative care improves survival in some patient populations. Several reasons could be invoked: avoidance of toxic nonbeneficial treatments, improved compliance with disease-directed treatments, and physiologic benefits resulting from effective symptom control (ie, relief of angina or dyspnea in patients with cardiomyopathy). In a 2007 study, the mean survival was 29 days longer for hospice patients than for nonhospice patients.[21] A recent study by Temel and colleagues[22] demonstrated early palliative care for patients with metastatic non-small–cell lung cancer is not only associated with significantly better quality of life, mood, and less aggressive treatment at end of life but also *increased survival*. Increased survival has been identified by Easson[23] as a potential outcome measure for palliative surgical procedures that had previously been recommended only for symptom control.

A significant factor in the rapid proliferation of hospital-based palliative care programs has no doubt been the cost avoidance realized by the reduction in hospital and ICU stays and costly invasive procedures resulting from effective palliative care team intervention. Not only has palliative care reduced hospital costs,[24] reduced days in the ICU and hospital,[25] it has also not been associated with increased mortality or morbidity. In some cases, the avoidance of invasive procedures that would have been performed on debilitated patients has probably increased their survival as well. The 30-day postoperative mortality and morbidity of patients with advanced cancer is considerable.[26] Despite these benefits, palliative care has not been timely[27] in the hospital setting.

Charles Von Gunten, currently Editor-in-Chief of *Palliative Medicine* and Chairman, Test Committee, Hospice and Palliative Medicine, American Board of Medical Specialties, and previous holder of many leadership positions in palliative care organizations, summarizes the change in palliative care over the past decade:

"To me, the most significant change is the move from palliative care as an 'option' or a 'choice' to proven gold standard of care that should be offered to all patients. We should be giving up any 'choice' language. It should all be focused now on 'how'." (Charles Von Gunten, MD, personal communication, September 9, 2010).

For an extensive and scholarly review of the growth and current status of palliative care in the United States, the reader is referred to Meier D. The development, status, and future of palliative care. In: Meier D, Isaacs SL, Hughes R, editors. Palliative care: transforming the care of serious illness. San Francisco: Jossey Bass; 2010. p. 1–464. Available at http://www.rwjf.org/files/research/4558.pdf.

See **Table 2** for a list of additional resources for surgeons interested in palliative care.

SURGERY AND PALLIATIVE CARE: THE ROLE OF THE AMERICAN COLLEGE OF SURGEONS

Over the past 15 years, the American College of Surgeons has been the primary catalyst for the recognition of palliative care in the field of surgery, primarily through educational efforts. The college has also endorsed palliative care in a series of professional standards statements[28,29] and public policy recommendations.[30] Much credit is due to the personal interest of the highest level of the college's leadership and its Division of Education, the sustained efforts of Wendy Husser who initiated the surgical palliative care series for the *Journal of the American College of Surgeons*, and Linn Meyer who never missed an opportunity to advocate for palliative care through her administration of public relations outlets for the college. During the past 2 decades, the college's perspective on end-of-life matters has evolved from debating physician-assisted suicide (PAS) in the mid to late 1990s to recognizing and implementing clinical approaches to palliative care in the current decade. No matter what position was taken in the physician-assisted suicide debate, it did little to improve symptom relief and clinical guidance for thousands of patients and families with life-limiting illness. In the late 1990s, most surgeons would have equated end-of-life care with hospice, PAS, or medical ethics. Since then, a broader understanding of the relevance of quality-of-life outcomes to day-to-day decision making and treatments for patients who are seriously ill has emerged. This understanding is reflected in 2 position statements of the college in 1998 and 2005. The first statement refers specifically to end of life and hospice, reinforcing the impression that palliative care is something that happens in the last stages of life. The subsequent statement is framed in language that adapts palliative principles to a much more broad population for whom death is not imminent or certain but for whom distress is likely, such as those in a critical care setting or with a new diagnosis of cancer. Currently, the college is focusing on

Table 2	
Palliative care education resources for surgeons	
Center to Advance Palliative Care Available at: http://www.capc.org/	The Center to Advance Palliative Care provides health care professionals with tools, training, and technical assistance necessary to start and sustain palliative care programs in hospitals and other health care settings.
Education of Physicians about End-of-Life Care Available at: http://www.eperc.mcw.edu/	This site has been designed for use by medical school course/clerkship directors, residency, and continuing education program directors, medical faculty, community preceptors, or other professionals who are (or will be) involved in providing end-of-life instruction to health care professionals in training.
Dunn G, Martensen R, Weissman D, editors. *Surgical palliative care: A resident's guide.* Chicago: American College of Surgeons. Cuniff-Dixon Foundation; 2009. Available through American College of Surgeons 633 N, St Clair Street Chicago, IL 60,611–3211	Guide introducing surgeons in training to the basic principles and practices of surgical palliative care
Hospice and Palliative Care Training for Physicians: UNIPAC, 3rd edition. American Academy of hospice and Palliative Medicine Available at: http://www.aahpm.org/ resources/default/training.html	9 module self-study program for physicians, which introduces hospice and palliative care concepts and practices for a variety of patient groups (cancer, chronic obstructive pulmonary disease, dementia, HIV/AIDS, pediatrics
Walsh D, Caraceni AT, Fainsinger R, et al, editors. *Palliative Medicine.* Philadelphia: Saunders-Elsevier; 2009.	Hardbound and online textbook of palliative medicine with contributions from many pioneers of the specialty

the education of surgeons and surgeons in training in the strategy and tactics of palliative care, communication, and symptom management (**Box 2**),[31] while not abandoning its long-standing attention to medical ethics.[32] A recent important contribution of the college's Commission on Cancer has been the addition of a new Cancer Program Standard for 2012 that states, "Palliative care services are available to patients on-site or by referral."[33]

To summarize the college's contribution to the evolution of surgical palliative care over the past 2 decades, it started with its search for an effective strategy for the care of patients at the end of life following the establishment of the legal pathway to freedom from futile or undesired treatments as laid out in the landmark cases of Quinlan[34] (ruling allowed withdrawal of ventilator support from patient in permanent vegetative state), Cruzan[35] (ruling affirmed that patients who could not make decisions still retained a right to refuse medical treatment), and its acknowledgment of end-of-life issues within the limited scope of the physician-assisted suicide debate. From the previous highly intellectualized ethical discourse evolved a more practical concern about how surgeons should communicate with patients who are seriously ill, how

---

Box 2
List of teaching modules in surgical palliative care: a resident's guide

- Personal awareness, self-care, and the surgeon-patient relationship
- Pain
- Dyspnea
- Delirium
- Depression
- Nausea
- Constipation
- Malignant bowel obstruction
- Cachexia, anorexia, asthenia, fatigue (wasting syndromes)
- Artificial nutrition and hydration
- Palliative surgery: definition, principles, outcomes assessment
- Pediatric palliative care
- Cross-cultural encounters
- Delivering bad news
- Goals of care/conducting a family conference
- The do not resuscitate discussion
- Palliative and hospice care referrals
- Care during the final days of life
- Discussing spiritual issues: maintaining hope

From Dunn G, Martensen R, Weissman D, editors. Surgical palliative care: a resident's guide. Chicago: American College of Surgeons. Cuniff-Dixon Foundation; 2009; with permission.

---

they should manage their most troubling symptoms, and how they can contribute to the restoration of hope using their own and their patients' personal, socioeconomic, and spiritual assets. Growing public interest and awareness of end-of-life issues and its implications for future health policy advocacy has catalyzed this transition.

PALLIATIVE CARE AND THE AMERICAN BOARD OF SURGERY

The American Board of Surgery was one of 10 boards of the American Board of Medical Specialties that sponsored the formation of the subspecialty of Hospice and Palliative Medicine in 2006. A small number of surgeons have been certified to date. Up until now 2 paths to certification have been open to surgeons seeking certification in hospice and palliative medicine: experiential and fellowship. The window for grandfathering is closing, as the required 2-year period of affiliation with a hospice or palliative care team has already started for those attempting to sit for the next (2012) examination. Following 2012, completion of an ACGME-credited palliative medicine fellowship program will be required to sit for the examination. Apart from offering a certification in hospice and palliative medicine, the American Board of Surgery considers palliative care skills among the expected domains of competence for surgeons seeking board certification.[36]

SURGICAL PALLIATIVE CARE ACROSS THE SPECTRUM OF SURGERY

Currently, the concept of surgical palliative care appears to be establishing itself in critical and trauma care mainly because of the similarities of palliative care and critical care as previously outlined. Access to palliative care in that setting is still quite limited and not improved by use of triggers to prompt palliative care referrals.[37] However, a recent presentation[38] at the American College of Surgeons' 96th Annual Clinical Congress demonstrated the compatibility of palliative care for transplantation patients in all stages of the transplantation continuum. In a recent study, trauma-burn surgeons and neurosurgeons reported being better equipped to manage multidimensional suffering of patients with sudden advanced illness when collaborating with a palliative care team.[39] Jacobs and colleagues[40] published a best-practice model for end-of-life support for trauma patients and their families. It stands as a model for the application of surgical palliative care in other venues beyond trauma care because it is a systems-based and interdisciplinary model. The American Trauma Society has published a valuable contribution to surgical palliative care in *The Second Trauma Program. The Art of Communicating with Families of Trauma Patients.*[41] The *second trauma* that the title refers to is the emotional trauma that happens to the family of the victim, the *first trauma* is the injury to the victim. The manual outlines communication and support techniques and strategies. It also addresses specific issues, such as family support after suicide, requests for organ donation, family presence during resuscitation, and suspected abuse.

The field of surgical oncology has seen a consensus and refinement of the definition of palliative surgery (see **Table 1**). The definition that has emerged is now in alignment with palliative as understood by the rest of the field of palliative care. Other contributions will include increased use of less invasive surgical techniques (see the article by Jay Requarth elsewhere in this issue for further exploration of this topic) and better prognostication, especially for those patients for whom operative intervention is being considered. A nomogram has recently been developed to predict 30-day morbidity and mortality for patients with disseminated malignancy undergoing surgical intervention.[42] This type of innovation will be a valuable adjunct to the developing field of communication. The social, ethical, and statistical complexity of designing clinical trials for palliative surgical outcomes[43,44] will benefit from the extensive experience and work that has been done in nonsurgical palliative care research.

SURGICAL PALLIATIVE CARE: WILL IT TRANSFORM SURGERY AND SURGEONS?

What will successful implementation of palliative care in the field of surgery look like? It will be successfully established when any surgical patient who is seriously ill and their family know to request palliative care; all surgeons have the willingness, knowledge, and skills to ensure their patients will receive palliative care; and the surgical venue will be prepared and equipped to provide palliative care. This success will require not only a change in the cognitive and technical repertoire of the surgeon but also a change of the surgical character that is willing to risk some degree of psychologic and spiritual reflection and introspection. In the past, surgeons have made similarly significant adjustments. The eighteenth century surgeon who relied on speed and callousness to accomplish life-saving amputations yielded to the more deliberate, cerebral, and gentler surgeon of the late nineteenth and twentieth century who performed reconstructions. It seems particularly appropriate in the current era of social networking and globalization to ask if the surgeon of the twenty-first century be noted for their ability to recognize the impact of their intervention beyond the merely physical aspects the patients' experience and its impact beyond the individual patient.

Palliative care is not care for the dying, but care of people with serious or life-limiting illness, some of whom will die imminently. To limit the concept of palliative care to the dying only reinforces the current Western dichotomous view of life and death, which could be summarized as all or nothing or fight or flight. The richness of palliative care lies in its recognition of the possible where there is uncertainty. There is nothing uncertain about robust health or active dying. This philosophy is an extension of the hospice philosophy that has facilitated the transition from *death as failure* to *dying as opportunity*. For those who actually are at the end of their life, palliative care offers the opportunity to die in peace instead of pieces. For those not at the end of life, palliative care offers the same hope: to live in peace, not piecemeal. The surgical world has too many seriously ill people in its care and has too much to offer the seriously ill with all diagnoses to not assume a leadership role for the continued growth and development of palliative care. Recent developments in the field of surgery give reason for optimism that this will occur.

REFERENCES

1. Dunn G. Surgical palliative care. In: Cameron J, editor. Current surgical therapy. 9th edition. Philadelphia: Mosby, Elsevier; 2008. p. 1179.
2. Clemens KE, Jaspers B, Klaschik E. The history of hospice. In: Walsh D, Caraceni AT, Fainsinger R, et al, editors. Palliative medicine. Philadelphia: Saunders-Elsevier; 2009. p. 20.
3. Available at: http://www.aahpm.org/certification/abms.html. Accessed September 12, 2010.
4. National Consensus Project for Quality Palliative Care. Clinical practice guidelines (2004). Available at: http://www.nationalconsensusproject.org/Guidelines_Download.asp. Accessed January 13, 2011.
5. National Quality Forum. A national framework and preferred practices for palliative and hospice care; December 2006. Available at: http://www.qualityforum.org/publications/reports/palliative.asp. Accessed January 13, 2011.
6. Bronner E. The foundation's end of life programs: changing the American way of death. To improve health and health care, vol. vi: the Robert Wood Johnson Foundation anthology. San Francisco (CA): Jossey-Bass; 2003.
7. McGlinchey L, editor. Transforming the culture of dying: the project on death in America, October 1994—December, 2003. New York: Open Society Institute; 2004. p. 1–72.
8. Poisal JA, Truffer C, Smith C, et al. Health spending projections through 2016: modest changes obscure part D's impacts. Health Aff 2007;26:W242–53.
9. Teno JM, Clarridge BR, Casey V, et al. Family perspectives on end-of-life care at the last place of care. JAMA 2004;291:88–93.
10. Center to Advance Palliative Care. National palliative care research center. America's care of serious illness: a state-by-state report card on access to palliative care in our nation's hospitals. Available at: http://www.capc.org/reportcard/state-by-state-report-card.pdf. Accessed, January 14, 2011.
11. Center to Advance Palliative Care. Palliative care NCP guidelines-center to advance palliative care. Available at: www.capc.org/ncp-guidelines/view?searchterm=clinical%20practice%20guidelines. Accessed January 14, 2011.
12. Office of Geriatrics and Extended Care. US department of veteran's affairs. hospice and palliative care. Available at: ww1.va.gov/GERIATRICS/Hospice_Palliative_Care2.asp. Accessed January 14, 2011.

13. Wall RJ, Curtis JR, Cooke CR, et al. Family satisfaction in the ICU: differences between families of survivors and nonsurvivors. Chest 2007;132(5):1425–33.

14. Curtis JR, White DB. Practical guidance for evidence-based ICU family conferences. Chest 2008;134(4):835–43.

15. Azoulay E, Pochard F, Kentish-Barnes N, et al. Risk of post-traumatic stress symptoms in family members of intensive care unit patients. Am J Respir Crit Care Med 2005;171(9):987–94.

16. Nelson JE, Bassett R, Boss RD, et al. Models for structuring a clinical initiative to enhance palliative care in the intensive care unit: a report from the IPAL-ICU Project (improving palliative care in the ICU). Crit Care Med 2010;38(9): 1765–72.

17. Higginson IJ, Finlay I, Goodwin DM, et al. Do hospital-based palliative teams improve care for patients or families at the end of life? J Pain Symptom Manage 2002;23:96–106.

18. Higginson IJ, Finlay IG, Goodwin DM, et al. Is there evidence that palliative care teams alter end-of-life experiences of patients and their caregivers? J Pain Symptom Manage 2003;25:150–68.

19. Finlay IG, Higginson IJ, Goodwin DM, et al. Palliative care in hospital, hospice, at home: results from a systematic review. Ann Oncol 2002;13(Suppl 4):257–64.

20. Casarett D, Pickard A, Bailey FA, et al. Do palliative care consultations improve patient outcomes? J Am Geriatr Soc 2008;56(4):593–9.

21. Connor SR, Pyenson B, Fitch K, et al. Comparing hospice and non-hospice patient survival among patients who die within a three year window. J Pain Symptom Manage 2007;33(3):238–46.

22. Temel JS, Greer JA, Muzikansky A, et al. Early palliative care for patients with metastatic non-small-cell lung cancer. N Engl J Med 2010;363(8):733–42.

23. Cady B, Barker F, Easson A. Part 3: surgical palliation of advanced illness: what's new, what's helpful. J Am Coll Surg 2005;200(3):457–66.

24. Penrod JD, Deb P, Dellenbaugh C, et al. Hospital-based palliative care consultation: effects on hospital cost. J Palliat Med 2010;13(8):973–9.

25. Ciemins EL, Blum L, Nunley M, et al. The economic and clinical impact of an inpatient palliative care consultation service. J Palliat Med 2007;10:1347–55.

26. Cady B, Miner T, Morgentaler A. Part 2: surgical palliation of advanced illness: what's new, what's helpful. J Am Coll Surg 2005;200(2):281–90.

27. Penrod JD, Deb P, Luhrs C, et al. Cost and utilization outcomes of patients receiving hospital-based palliative care consultation. J Palliat Med 2006;9(4): 855–60. [erratum in: J Palliat Med 2006;9(6):1509].

28. American College of Surgeons Committee on Ethics. Statement of principles guiding care at the end of life. Bull Am Coll Surg 1998;83(4):46.

29. American College of Surgeons Committee on Ethics and Surgical Palliative Care Task Force. Statement of principles of palliative care. Bull Am Coll Surg 2005; 90(8):34–45.

30. American College of Surgeons. Statement on health care reform. Bull Am Coll Surg 2008;93:1–5.

31. Dunn G, Martensen R, Weissman D, editors. Surgical palliative care: a resident's guide. American college of surgeons. Chicago: Cuniff-Dixon Foundation; 2009. p. 107–32.

32. McGrath MH, Risucci DA, Schwab A, editors. Ethical issues in clinical surgery. Chicago: American College of Surgeons; 2007. p. 1–149.

33. Commission on Cancer. Cancer Program Standards 2012. American College of Surgeons. Chicago, in press.

34. In Re Quinlan, 355 A.2d 647 (N.J. 1976).
35. Cruzan v Missouri Department of Health, 497 U.S. 261 (1990).
36. Available at: http://home.absurgery.org/xfer/BookletofInfo-Surgery.pdf. Accessed January 13, 2011.
37. Bradley C, Weaver J, Brasel K. Addressing access to palliative care services in the surgical intensive care unit. Surgery 2010;147(6):871–7.
38. Aloia TA. Syndrome of imminent demise. Panel session 219: common problems and quality outcomes: surgical care for the terminal patient. American College of Surgeons 96th Annual Clinical Congress. Washington, DC, October 5, 2010.
39. Tilden LB, Williams BR, Tucker RO, et al. Surgeons' attitudes and practices in the utilization of palliative and supportive care services for patients with a sudden advanced illness. Palliat Med 2009;12(11):1037–42.
40. Jacobs BB, Jacobs LM, Burns K. Trauma end of life optimum support. A best practice model for trauma professionals. Woodbury (CT): CineMed Publishing, Inc; 2010. p. 1–127.
41. Cronin M, Kelly P, Lipton, et al. The 2nd trauma program. The art of communicating with families of trauma patients. Upper Marlboro (MD): American Trauma Society; 2006. p. 1–50.
42. Tseng WH, Yang XY, Wang H, et al. Nomogram to predict risk of 30-day morbidity and mortality for patients with disseminated malignancy undergoing surgical intervention. Presented at the American Society of Clinical Oncology Annual Meeting. Chicago, June 4–8, 2010.
43. Mularski RA, Rosenfeld K, Coons SJ, et al. Measuring outcomes in randomized prospective trials in palliative care. J Pain Symptom Manage 2007;34(Suppl 1): S7–19.
44. Krouse RS, Easson AM, Angelos P. Ethical considerations and barriers to research in surgical palliative care. J Am Coll Surg 2003;196(3):469–74.
45. National Consensus Project. Clinical practice guidelines for quality palliative care. 2009. Available at: www.nationalconsensusproject.org. Accessed September 12, 2010.
46. Doyle D, Hanks G, Cherny N, et al. Introduction. In: Doyle D, Hanks G, Cherny N, et al, editors. Oxford textbook of palliative medicine, 3rd edition. Oxford (UK): Oxford University Press; 2004. p. 1.

Are Surgeons Capable of Introspection?

David W. Page, MD

KEYWORDS

- Introspection • Self-reflection • Surgical personality • Empathy
- Palliative surgery

The philosophy of the wisest man that ever existed is mainly derived from the act of introspection.

William Godwin

Think of introspection as just another "time out." Perhaps surgeons would feel better working from a checklist of exploratory questions to ask when thinking about their thoughts and actions? Surgeons might consider introspection a cognitive "operation" that requires planning. And, of course, there are risks to the process of digging around in one's mind uncovering notions about good and evil and the role of chance and uncertainty in one's practice and life.

Risks, benefits, and outcomes rule the surgical ethos. In the domain of palliative care, where a confrontation with one's own mortality is unavoidable, these elements may be seen as the core of introspection. When one considers the ramifications of the action-oriented "surgical personality," it becomes apparent that self-reflection may be anathema to some practitioners. Both surgeons and non-surgeons have written extensively about surgical personality traits and how they may impact the way surgeon's conduct their work.[1–6] This article probes the underbelly of what most observers agree is a unique surgical persona and discusses how it confounds the act of introspection.

In his insightful 1995 memoir, *A Miracle and a Privilege*, Francis D. Moore[7] wrote regarding end of life care, "Responsible physicians should join forces with the public to write a new chapter in medical education that places care in death in its proper context. It is tricky. It is dangerous. We need it and people are ready for it. It will relieve more suffering than did the discovery of anesthesia 150 years ago." Insight distilled from a lifetime of research and practice sparkle throughout Dr Moore's book, a repository of knowledge that not surprisingly includes the above quote referring to palliative care as part of a surgeon's responsibilities. Other physicians have also been aware of the need for self-reflection to understand the impact of their professional deeds on

No financial disclosures.

Department of Surgery, Tufts University School of Medicine, Baystate Medical Center, 759 Chestnut Street, Springfield, MA 01199, USA

E-mail address: david.page@bhs.org

patients. In discussing the need for self-awareness, Timothy Quill[8] wrote, "Unfortunately, most physicians are given little encouragement or training in looking inside themselves and exploring potential sources of strong reactions and identifications. In fact, there may frequently be a conspiracy to suppress such reactions in the belief that they should not exist in a 'professional' physician-patient relationship." Subverting one's strong personal feelings in the service of helping others may, at first, seem unquestionably altruistic. Yet, a failure to understand one's own emotions could over time culminate in resentment and anger toward patients, emotions that can easily spill into the clinical encounter. Quill added, "A truly self-aware clinician will be able to determine if the source of a strong reaction is the clinician him- or herself, the patient, or the interaction of the two."[8] And as one might suspect, this issue is not new. In 1923, Deaver and Reimann[9] wrote, "Complacency and smug satisfaction are danger signals of decadence, just as wholesome discontent and healthy introspection and self-criticism are indications of the will and desire for improvement."

Challenges offered by the current surgical environment as well as the impact of the surgical personality will influence a surgeon's willingness to include palliative care as an important aspect of his or her practice. However, to do so will no doubt nudge us away from the danger signals of decadence.

CHALLENGES OF THE TWENTY-FIRST CENTURY SURGICAL ENVIRONMENT

Both academic surgeons and private practitioners face enormous challenges today. The litany of issues runs a familiar course from a surgeon shortage, reduced reimbursement, mounting clinical work, cognitive and technical overload secondary to minimally invasive surgery superimposed upon traditional open techniques, a severe reduction in trainee duty hours and the consequent educational dilemmas, and oppressive regulatory oversight. Getting the work done safely and efficiently is time-consuming. Few moments remain at the end of the day for self-reflection. One might worry that too much introspection could be harmful. I will argue that without regular self-assessment a surgeon may fall into the trap of depression, substance abuse, or full-blown burnout.

Surgeons have always paid a price for their dedication to the ideal of providing the personal continuity of care they feel is a unique aspect of the management of operative patients. The result of this self-imposed burden is fatigue and frustration. Only 75% of surgeons recently surveyed stated that they enjoy the practice of surgery and 30% to 40% suffered from burnout.[10] This syndrome is characterized by depersonalization and a loss of interest in one's patients, as well as in the performance of the technical work itself. Not only are these surgeons a threat to their patients' safety, they also risk the consequences of burnout, namely poor clinical performance, divorce, and alcoholism.[11] Paradoxically, becoming more rather than less involved with sick patients could provide an opportunity for surgeons to explore their feelings and views about death and other end-of-life issues. The overwhelming impact of a confrontation with a dying patient often serves to place one's own day-to-day conundrums in perspective. Measuring one's good fortune against the faltering final steps of another human being seems to me to be life's ultimate metric.

Thus, my argument is that surgeons who routinely abandon their dying patients to the care of others have not only tossed away an opportunity to help their patients accomplish the chores of dying, but they have also lost an opportunity to cultivate self-knowledge. Some surgeons may not feel comfortable talking to dying patients. However, at least one study refutes this tenacious allegation.[12] Too often palliative surgical care is viewed as a matter of operative intervention, the employment of procedures designed to relieve suffering. That aspect of a surgeon's work with the dying is important, but operating at the end of life is only a part of how they may help patients with incurable disease.

THE VARIABLE ENDOWMENT OF REFLECTIVE THOUGHT—LEVELS OF CARING

Not all surgeons limit themselves by adhering to the constrained professional paradigm referred to as the "action as success" principle. In fact, many academic and community surgeons frequently reflect on the challenges of their surgical practices with genuine insight. To be fair to the others, busy practitioners have little time to reflect on their daily actions—excluding the painful soul-searching all surgeons indulge in when complications arise. For some practitioners the notion of looking inward is both rewarding and troublesome. It is for precisely this reason that surgeons would benefit from taking moments here and there to consider the weight of their work, particularly when it involves terminally sick patients.

Daniel Callahan[13] describes four levels of potential involvement in patient care. These categories may serve as a framework for surgeons to determine how deeply to get involved when asked to participate in a particular patient's care. Callahan writes derisively about modern medicine's preoccupation with cure, "For its part, scientific medicine seems to have said that it is not its task to understand and give meaning to suffering but to rid our lives of it. Meaning, like caring, is for the losers."[13] In contrast to employing a purely scientific biomedical model of patient management, caring surgeons may become truly engaged in their patient's care by encouraging an ongoing dialog to explore the patient's hopes and fears about dying.

Imagine that a surgeon has been asked to consult on an elderly jaundiced patient with a forty-pound weight loss and an epigastric mass. Suspecting an inoperable pancreatic cancer, he or she summon up a snapshot overview of what may be going on with the patient and where the relentless clinical course will go. The surgeon's involvement will be easier to formulate if the consult is framed with the following levels of possible interaction in mind[2]:

- Cognitive involvement (providing one's assessment of the diagnosis and the patient's treatment options)
- Emotional involvement (acknowledging the patient's fear, anxiety, dread, etc)
- Values (making certain one understands that his or her values and what the patient believes is important may differ)
- Relationships (Is the patient open to the opinions of others? To the surgeon's opinion? Does the surgeon know the family members and what they think?)

The surgeon's opinion regarding the choice of a biliary or gastric bypass, or neither, as well as other operative possibilities is the cognitive element of the consult. The discussion may be suffused with the patient's (and the surgeon's) anxieties regarding the threat of shortening the patient's life as a consequence of postoperative complications, as well as the patient's values regarding how hard to fight. And the family may enter the consultation dialog and deepen the surgeon's involvement. Thus, a surgical consult may be singularly focused on the wisdom of surgical intervention or may become intimate and ongoing.

DOES THE SURGICAL PERSONALITY EXCLUDE INTROSPECTION?

Three well-known anthropologists as well as a number of surgeons have studied and recorded what are perceived to be the primary elements of a surgical personality.

Some observers have debated the existence of personality traits specific to surgeons, but most agree surgeons share common thinking habits and behavior patterns (stereotypical responses) in given situations. This article highlights the contributions of Charles Bosk, Joan Cassell, Pearl Katz, and other investigators who have delineated the characteristics felt to be typical of the surgeons they observed or surveyed. This information emerged from the 1970s and 1980s. When blended with more recent contributions from surgeons themselves, it constitutes timeless insight into the workings of the surgical mind and will inform this discussion of introspection.

Long before Henry the VIII directed the creation of the Company of Barber Surgeons in London in 1540, physicians and surgeons had separated themselves from one another along elitist and intellectual lines. Surgeons were uneducated and crude, yet increasingly effective at managing superficial surgical diseases such as abscesses, fractures, dislocations, and wounds. The origins of surgery reflect the very antithesis of introspection. With anesthesia far in the future, cutting for bladder stones and excising surface tumors were operations attempted by skilled surgeons employing personal courage, as well as alcoholic beverages and sedative nostrums, for their luckless patients. Before ether, nitrous oxide, and chloroform, surgeons made their reputations by demonstrating remarkable hand speed.

The modern era of surgery with its advances in surgical techniques, as well as improved pre- and postoperative care, has eliminated the need for "prima donna" boldness and sheer extroversion. Joan Cassell[2] reminds us of the reluctantance to stereotype or label members of society even though she describes in detail specific traits of the surgeons she studied. As recently as three decades ago, trainees were inured to, "Be ballsy. Do it!" following in the footsteps of their male mentors (and ridiculing women who dared to enter the male-dominated cloister of surgeons).[14]

In her 1991 book, *Expected Miracles—surgeons at work*, Cassell wrote regarding heroic curing versus healing illness, "Heroes ignore patients' subjective experiences of being unwell, unfit. Patients suffering from illness are frequently labeled 'complainers' by heroic surgeons who knowing they excised disease, resent the patient's unabated demand for care."[14] In the surgical world of the 1970s and 1980s, surgeons described themselves to Cassell as "macho" lovers of sports and cars, acting as if invulnerable, untiring, and fearless. She noted similarities between surgeons and test pilots, both masculine worlds of death-defying activities, long training periods, and high levels of technical skills. She also noted the following surgical personality traits: arrogance, certitude, activism, and qualities of strong leadership.

Thus, Cassell articulates the dilemma at the center of this discussion: "It may be the exceptional surgeon who is capable of recognizing and supporting the autonomy of patients, of allowing them to share decision-making, of acknowledging uncertainty in the face of decisions that must be made. Such people surely exist, but perhaps we cannot expect them to be the temperamental or behavioral norm among surgeons."[14] Why not? Should surgeons not expect more of themselves in today's complex health care environment? If surgeons do not participate fully in their patients care, do they not feed the old prejudice of "surgeon-as-technician"?

Cassell wrote elsewhere of the surgeon's personality traits, "As for sympathy, empathy, and an aptitude for human relations, these traditionally female traits seem somewhat peripheral to the most obvious and easily observed characteristics of a good surgeon, many of which are exhibited when the patient is unconscious."[2] She concludes that, because surgery is a public act, the surgeon's relationship with disease is personal; surgical success is *attributable* (to the surgeon's skill) and *visible* (in the operating room).

Pearl Katz's[15] 1990 book, *The Scalpel's Edge*, is a rich trove of observations from her study of a large North American teaching hospital in the 1980s. She observed surgeons in action as well as documented their attitudes regarding their work, trainees, and peers. She noted that surgeons focus on the mechanical repair of the body in a hospital setting that fragments care (rounds aimed at specific postoperative goals) and provides scant opportunity for the surgeon to become intimately acquainted with his or her patients. Referring to the often unpleasant visceral nature of surgery, Katz writes, "Surgeon's detachment from their patients may be understood as necessary protections for these routine sights, smells, acts, and dramatic confrontations with mortality.... It may be that if a surgeon were to empathize with each of his patients who are in fear, pain, and confusion and are sick and dying, his efficacy as a surgeon may be compromised."[15] Therein lies the rub for all who walk the invisible line between necessary detachment and appropriate intimacy with patients.

However, the skilled surgeon ought to be able to step away from the bright operating room lights, away from the invisible patient beneath the drapes—the dictates of sterility having removed any visible evidence of the humanity in the room—and later sit at the patient's bedside and indulge in the empathetic exchange that postoperative patients seek. Commenting on surgeons' tendency to boldly rebuff uncertainty, Katz states, "Thinking that emphasizes certainty diverges considerably from (scientific) thinking which emphasizes skepticism, questioning, knowledge-seeking, reflection, analysis, and verification."[15]

In the 1980s, surgeons favored action over cerebration. And, when debating clinical issues among themselves, surgeons for the better part of the twentieth century preferred heated exchanges, if not outright acrimonious dialog in discussing clinical trials and scientific data. Katz[15] noted that the surgeons she observed expressed several traits including impatience, ill-disguised condescension, mild distrust, need for positive feedback about their performances, insistence on an unequal distribution of power, and secretiveness manifested as a poor ability to communicate with their colleagues. The image of the surgeon as masculine hero evolved to its highest form through the last decade of the twentieth century; war metaphors punctuated the surgical lexicon then and they continue to find their way into the language of lay people today. For example, obituaries refer to the inevitability of metastatic disease as "losing the battle with cancer." The language of surgeons often includes references to "conquests," "victories over disease," "patient's defenses," and "taking the offensive against disease" by "heroes" and "warriors" who show courage through action. Thus, Katz[15] concludes, "They reveal their proclivity for action in their use of language which not only prefers using active words and active tense, but also refers to battles and wars, strength and masculinity, while denigrating weakness, passivity, and femininity."

This language hardly reflects the temperament of individuals inclined to practice introspection.

It is unclear how thoroughly today's surgeons have discarded the traditional heroic stature Katz and Cassell observed and described. It is not only a matter of how the world at large envisions their work and general conduct; the issue also revolves around how surgeons view themselves. It is my sense that the heroic "militaristic" persona of surgeons has been modified and diluted by two recent advances: the entry of more women into surgery and the very different demands of minimally invasive surgery. Together, these two changes may significantly improve palliative surgical care.

In 1999, Ronald M. Epstein[16] wrote in *JAMA*, "Exemplary physicians seem to have a capacity for critical self-reflection that pervades all aspects of practice, including being present with the patient, solving problems, eliciting and transmitting information, making evidence-based decisions, performing technical skills, and defining their own values." By the end of the decade of the 1990s, minimally invasive surgery had changed the radical nature of operations and had similarly begun to modulate the surgeon's image. Instruments and incisions had become smaller and hand delicacy proved to be even more essential than with open operations. Today, just as less tissue trauma continues to be of paramount importance, surgeons have been brought to adhere to strict behavioral standards. Managing conflict represents another nontechnical skill required of today's surgical practitioners.[17]

One wonders if the traditional surgical personality will become obsolete.

DOES PATIENT AUTONOMY IMPROVE WITH SURGEON INTROSPECTION?

Choice remains at the heart of end-of-life decisions. The World Health Organization has emphasized the view that palliative care encompasses the total care of patients whose disease is not responsive to any curative treatment.[18] It is the inability to accept the value of caring over the value of curing that often turns surgeons away from playing a role in the final chapter of their patient's life. Despite discussions to the contrary, surgeons continue to view death as defeat—just as they interpret the need to open during a laparoscopic case as a crushing blow to their egos. Neither sentiment is appropriate, although not unexpected from highly motivated practitioners. The often repeated expression about surgeons, "Sometimes wrong, but never in doubt," serves to highlight the issue: without a sense of self-doubt there is often little room in patient-surgeon communication for considering options, for choice, and for patient autonomy.

Thus, the two ideas being discussed often clash in the surgeon's mind with the arrival of a need for palliation—the notion of patient autonomy versus the surgeon's self-image as leader and action hero. Accustomed to directing patient care in the operating room and, to a lesser degree, in the office or clinic, surgeons may well step back in annoyance from patients who express a desire to be autonomous in matters of end-of-life care. To appreciate the difficulty surgeons may have with end-of-life care, they must compare the long-standing tradition of the surgeon's self-image as action professional with other physicians' efforts to foster personal awareness. For example, Longhurst[19] emphasizes the need for doctors to understand how to see themselves as reflected in their patients' responses to them, as well as the imperative to understand the impact on patients of the doctor's subjective internal world of beliefs, values, attitudes and fantasies. Without self-knowledge, the surgeon may mistake his or her treatment choices for those of the patient.

Surgeons would do well to review the dysfunctional beliefs held by many doctors (convictions too often taken to heart by surgeons) as articulated by Martin[20]: (1) high physician expectations make the limitations of one's knowledge a personal failure, (2) responsibility for patient care is to be borne by physicians alone, (3) altruistic devotion to one's work and denial of self is desirable, and (4) it is professional to keep one's uncertainties and emotions to oneself. These destructive and closely held beliefs are nothing if not a recipe for burnout. Other topics surgeons should consider for self-review as well as discussion with one's peers include gender issues, one's feelings and reactions to difficult patients, anger management, boundary issues, and personal bias about certain types of patients (eg, AIDS patients, alcoholics, the homeless). Understanding one's anger is particularly important. Novak and colleagues[21] state, in an article on personal awareness, "Self-knowledge about the sources and triggers of one's anger and attitudes and skills related to conflict are particularly important because anger is a common response to illness, suffering, and death."

Anthropologist Charles Bosk[22] studied surgeons on the West Coast in the 1970s. Regarding the attitude of surgical trainees being inculcated into the "culture of surgeons" at that time, he concluded, "They treat all repressive sanctions as flowing from the arbitrary, capricious, dogmatic, and unreasonably autocratic personalities of attendings rather than from deeply held common sentiments shared by a community of fellow surgeons…. All shortcomings become attributable to personality and style." Bosk reiterated the view that a surgeon's unbridled optimism and certainty may serve as a form of denial about the possibility of failure. Katz reinforced this view that a scalpel-rattling posture by surgeons forces patients into a more passive role and thus reduces the likelihood of shared decision-making.

Similarly, surgeons have traditionally criticized other physicians for their contemplative demeanor, often portraying internists as procrastinators who may compromise the surgeon's conviction that "a chance to cut is a chance to cure." In 1923, Deaver and Reimann wrote, "…we daily have in our power to be the means of correcting mistakes in the interpretation of the language of living pathology, and thus save an otherwise condemned sufferer from medical procrastination."[9] Is it really procrastination? Or is it introspection? This sort of historically perpetuated surgical certainty (dare I call it hubris?) and the impulse for action—even though it is absolutely necessary at times—can only be subdued with honest self-examination.

The issue at hand, then, is whether or not surgeons have evolved to a professional station compatible with introspection. Without introspection, surgeons are unlikely to overcome their penchant for control and domination of patients as well as trainees. Yet, there is reason to be hopeful. The fact that McCahill and colleagues,[12] who reported that surgeons surveyed in 2002 did not consider the avoidance of dying patients to be an issue, also revealed that the two biggest ethical dilemmas in surgical oncology were providing honest information without destroying hope and preserving patient choice. Certainly, this report suggests that the surveyed surgeons had engaged in self-reflection and had willingly confronted these major barriers to the provision of palliative care (in contrast to the paternal attitude noted in years past by anthropologists).

THE SURGEON'S DILEMMA—THE ALLURE OF THE MECHANICAL

Laparoscopic surgery has not only added impersonal physical distance between the surgeon and the patient, it has generated a new industry dedicated to making interesting instruments and miniature cameras and TV screens that illuminate and expose a new surgical environment. Minimally invasive surgery is a magnificent technical tour de force. Robots add to biomechanical proficiency as well as to the geography of indifference. Using a robotic operating system, the surgeon sits across from the patient and manipulates remote control "arms" that direct delicate instruments in the patient's belly, pelvis, or chest on the far side of the room. And, of course, the marginally absurd extension of this robotic event is telesurgery, in which the patient lies in a hospital across the nation or on the far side of the ocean from the operator. Clearly, there are reasonable applications for remote surgical technology. However, under these circumstances the patient-physician relationship is further burdened with the potential for poor communication.

Not that the traditional open operations are any less technical or less manufactured. Staplers come with variable loads, reticulated handles, and anvils requiring special expertise and attention to detail. Intracorporeal suturing and knot-tying have added to the modern surgeon's technical skills. And with 121 "essential" operations to learn,[23] the surgical trainee discovers the impossibility of mastering both open and minimally invasive operations in 5 years of training. Rather than the 10,000 hours of deliberate practice recommended by Ericsson and colleagues[24] when mastering chess or a musical instrument, surgical residents average between 1,100 and 2,700 hours of actual operating time.[25,26] Hence, surgical educators have become understandably preoccupied with the issue of technical competence at a time when the sheer number of operations available to the public is unmanageable by any single surgeon.

When are surgeons and trainees supposed to reflect on and master the nuances of palliative surgical care? There is only one answer. The attitude of caring in conjunction with curing must be ever-present on the front burner of surgical education. Caring must be modeled by the faculty. Insights gained from introspection by the teaching faculty should be shared with residents and medical students because almost 40% of residents in a recent study felt inadequately trained to discuss with their patients the withholding or withdrawal of life-sustaining therapy.[27] Surgeons must learn to be open with their intimate thoughts about caring for dying patients and seek opportunities to reveal themselves in their encounter with their learners.

SURGEON SELF-REFLECTION ENCOURAGES PATIENT'S SELF-STORY

A fact and a story when set next to each other ignite and illuminate the notion that, when encouraged to speak freely, patients flood the therapeutic encounter with meaning. The eighteen seconds that pass before a doctor interrupts his or her patient when taking a history,[28] stands in stark contrast to Rita Charon's[29] story of the man who burst into tears when given a chance to tell his illness story. No one had listened to him before his visit to her clinic. Charon concludes, "...not only is diagnosis encoded in the narratives patients tell of symptoms, but deep and therapeutically consequential understandings of the persons who bear symptoms are made possible in the course of hearing the narratives told of illness." Herein lies the severest challenge for surgeons whose personalities push them toward action, intervention, and instant discovery of solutions. Often the patient's personal narrative melts like ice cubes when the surgeon's blowtorch queries about the medical history narrow the focus to establishing a diagnosis. Rather than initially attempting to gain an understanding of the patient's perspective (dread, anxiety, fears) about the illness, the surgeon's "wired" clinical aggressiveness may set a tone of paternalism that shrinks the resolve of even the most autonomy-minded patient.

Limited time for each clinical encounter is the reality that frustrates an unimpeded verbal exchange between surgeon and patient. Nonetheless, even if it means another office visit or returning to the bedside at the end of the day, the patient must be given an opportunity to express his or her thoughts about possible treatment options versus no therapy. A patient who has received bad news must be given time to assimilate the life-changing information, to express fears and hopes, as well as to ask questions to expand his or her understanding of the prognosis. An introspective surgeon will share his or her carefully thought out concerns and will acknowledge and reflect the emotions in the room. By opening up the dialog and allowing the patient to indulge in his or her illness narrative, surgeons may discover ways around what moments earlier seemed like insurmountable barriers in defining the next step in the patient's care. By encouraging an open discussion regarding treatment options, the restrained (listening) surgeon may hear useful (as well as meaningful) dialog from the patient that brings the patient closer to moments of self-discovery and insight into the meaning of the illness.

Caring by the surgeon after the scalpel's job is done should continue long after curing proves futile. Part of the physician's job is to encourage the patient near the end of his or her life to do the sometimes strained work of dying—to settle emotional accounts with friends and family, to finalize personal and financial matters, and to reflect on the meaning of their life and death. This art must be taught as well. Thus, when talking to surgical residents and medical students about end of life care, faculty members are encouraged to model self-reflection and to share their own emotional reactions to the cases under discussion. Teachers are asked to encourage the trainee's own personal reflection by asking the following questions: (1) what is most challenging about working with this patient and family, (2) what is most satisfying about working with this patient and family (3) how is the trainee reacting emotionally to this patient, and (4) have the trainee's past experiences in any way enhanced or hindered his or her work with this patient and family?[30]

IRONIC SUFFERING AND A LACK OF INTROSPECTION

Sometimes a surgeon fails to exhibit "situational awareness." It starts with insensitivity—a failure to see the actual person behind the bandages or under the drapes. Usually, surgeons deal with their patients holistically from a physiologic point of view. This entails attention to fluid and electrolyte status, blood volume, wound care, urine output, oral intake, and so forth. It is a lot to review with every patient on the list—especially if the institution supports fast-tracking. The surgeon can easily fail to notice the emotional state of the person lying there, terrified, assuming the cancer operation did not work because the surgical team does not discuss the patient's real issue: "Am I going to make it?" Imagine the following communication imbroglio:

> Did you get it all, Doctor?
> The procedure went very smoothly, you know…technically.
> When will you get the path report?
> I expect you'll be home before it arrives…that's how well you're doing.
> Will I need chemo?
> We have a terrific group of medical oncologists here. I'm going to refer you to
>   my favorite. She'll answer all of your questions, believe me.
> But… Doctor, the cancer…
> Gone, the operation was a piece of cake.

Ivan Illyich had a busy family who failed to acknowledge his desperate plight. Of course to give his family their due, Ivan Illyich did everything humanly possible to deny his clinical symptoms until the very last moment. In the novella, *The Death of Ivan Illyich* (essential reading for anyone involved in palliative care), Tolstoy[31] bores deeply into the soul of a desperate man to reveal the secret anguish the dying experience while still among the living. And although Ivan Illyich brought his self-serving and aloof persona to his deathbed, he had to travel an unimaginable psychic distance in the act of dying to discover a fundamental human truth. As his life slipped away, Ivan Illyich's family went about their lives as if he were doing quite well. The crisp story defines ironic suffering. No one in his family would discuss his illness with him in a meaningful way. No one would acknowledge that Ivan Illyich was, in fact, dying before their eyes.

ARE WOMEN SURGEONS BETTER AT INTROSPECTION THAN MALE SURGEONS?

The short courageous history of women entering the ranks of surgery in the 1970s and 1980s (as documented in several enlightening books) reads like a portrayal of surgeons as abusive husbands.[2,15,32,33] At every turn men derided, discouraged, and humiliated women attempting to become competent surgeons. What is remarkable about this unimaginable resistance to change is, ironically, the old saw which is said to have originated with John Bell who, in describing the ideal surgeon, suggested he possess, "The brain of an Apollo, the heart of a lion, a clear eye, and a woman's touch."[34]

My experience with talented female surgical residents reinforces my conviction that they can function at any level on the male macho "toughness" scale while preserving inveterate empathy for their patients. As caregivers for everyone from children to grandparents, women have always shown unique insight into guardianship. Clearly, women have carried the burden of caring for elderly parents while a majority of them held fulltime jobs and managed a family. How could men believe that women would not make exceptional surgeons? With the waning of the surgical personality and, perhaps, if they listen, men may learn, standing at the side of women surgeons, the lessons and rewards residing in the domain of introspection. It seems certain that in the early days of female surgical resident training, male mentors lured women away from their natural self-reflective instincts and toward male indifference.

INTROSPECTION AT THE END OF A SURGEON'S CAREER

At this juncture, my thoughts drift to a consideration of a parallel course between the end of a surgeon's career with the termination of a patient's life. As when confronting death, completing a professional life ought to include the hard work of closure. The "tidying up" process at the end of a productive career requires no less intellectual and emotional diligence than that of the closure necessary for the dying. And, in fact, the events of these two seemingly disparate life events may overlap.

Offering thanks to family members and colleagues (as well as apologies for past "incidents") may be just as satisfying for a retiring surgeon as receiving empathetic words and closure are for a dying patient. In other words, the overarching opportunities dangling before the retiring surgeon are similar to the opportunities presented to a dying person—namely that of accomplishing life's final goals. The surgeon who has reflected on his or her professional and personal existence as an essential part of a life well lived will not have difficulty defining the goals of retirement. Among these goals might be involvement in surgical education, especially discussing end-of-life issues with residents. With the surgeon's own demise squarely located in the gauzy distance of retirement, the seasoned clinician possesses a unique perspective on life that medical students and residents are rarely exposed to in their training.

Not infrequently surgeons retire only to return to part-time work either in their former offices or in some administrative or teaching capacity at their hospital. Certainly there are many surgeons who will have planned properly for retirement and will slip without a ripple into the well-deserved and comforting waters of self-indulgence. But, some surgeons who might otherwise have been labeled with attention-deficit/hyperactivity disorder before it became fashionable, still find meaning in continuing to caring for patients and in teaching tomorrow's doctors as age creeps up.

The time for introspection is at the beginning of a career, not at the end. The habit of introspection may serve to enrich a surgeon's career with insight, as well as inform the empathetic care needed by cured and dying patients alike. And much like "the second effect" of opioid administration, although the intent of self-reflection is to improve patient care, the foreseen but unpredictable second consequence of introspection may be the arrival of profound insight into the meaning of one's life.

SUMMARY

The traditional action-oriented surgical personality, although essential in the service of solving emergent operative dilemmas, may serve as a barrier to introspection.

Certainly, challenges of the twenty-first century practice environment, not the least of which are time constraints, also distract from self-reflection. Without engaging in moments of introspection, surgeons risk not only abandoning dying patients in their time of need, but leave the surgeons themselves at risk for burnout and its dire consequences. The increase in the number of women in surgery, as well as the less heroic image of surgeons performing laparoscopic operations, may reorient traditional extroverted behavior toward a persona of professional grace.

REFERENCES

1. Greenburg AG, McClure MA, Penn NE. Personality traits of surgical house officers: faculty and resident views. Surgery 1982;92(2):368–72.
2. Cassell J. On control, certitude, and the "paranoia" of surgeons. Cult Med Psychiatry 1987;11:229–49.
3. Gordin R, Jacobsen SJ, Rimm AA. Similarities in the personalities of women and men who were first year medical students planning careers in surgery. Acad Med 1991;66(9):560.
4. Schwartz RW, Barclay JR, Harrell P, et al. Defining the surgical personality: a preliminary study. Surgery 1994;115:62–8.
5. Thomas JH. The surgical personality: fact or fiction. Am J Surg 1997;174:573–7.
6. McGreevy J, Wiebe D. A preliminary measurement of the surgical personality. Am J Surg 2002;184:121–5.
7. Moore FD. Ethics at both ends of life. In: A miracle and a privilege—recounting a half century of surgical advance. Washington, DC: Joseph Henry Press; 1995. p. 344.
8. Quill T. Humanistic end-of-life care. In: Caring for patients at the end of life: facing an uncertain future together. Oxford (UK): Oxford University Press; 2001. p. 25, 26.
9. Deaver JB, Reimann SP. Medical education and educators. In: Excursions into surgical subjects. Philadelphia: W.B. Saunders Company; 1923. p. 115, 161.
10. Balch CM, Freischlag JA, Shanafelt TA. Stress and burnout among—understanding and managing the syndrome and avoiding the adverse consequences. Arch Surg 2009;144(4):371–6.
11. Campbell DA, Sonnad SS, Eckhauser FE, et al. Burnout among American surgeons. Surgery 2001;130:696–705.
12. McCahill LE, Krouse RS, Chu DZ, et al. Decision making in palliative care. J Am Coll Surg 2002;195:411–23.
13. Callahan D. Our need for caring—vulnerability and illness. In: The lost art of caring: a challenge to health professionals, families, communities, and society. Baltimore (MD): The Johns Hopkins University Press; 2001. p. 14, 20–2.
14. Cassell J. The temperament of surgeons. In: Expected miracles—surgeons at work. Philadelphia: Temple University Press; 1991. p. 30, 33, 59.
15. Katz P. The scalpel's edge. Boston: Allyn and Bacon; 1999. p. vii–viix, 21, 51.
16. Epstein RM. Mindful practice. JAMA 1999;282(4):833.
17. Rogers DA, Lingard L. Surgeons managing conflict: a framework for understanding the challenge. J Am Coll Surg 2006;203(4):568–73.
18. Dunn GP. The surgeon and palliative care—an evolving perspective. Surg Oncol Clin N Am 2001;10(1):7–24.
19. Longhurst M. Physician self-awareness: the neglected insight. CMAJ 1988;139: 121–4.
20. Martin AR. Stress in residency: a challenge to personal growth. J Gen Intern Med 1986;1:252–7.

21. Novak DH, Suchman AL, Clark W, et al. Calibrating the physician: personal awareness and effective patient care. JAMA 1997;278:502–9.
22. Bosk C. Conclusion. In: Forgive and remember—managing medical failure. Chicago: The University of Chicago Press; 1979. p. 187.
23. Bell RH. Why Johnny cannot operate. Surgery 2009;146(4):533–42.
24. Ericsson KA, Krampe RT, Tesch-Romer C. The role of deliberate practice in the acquisition of expert performance. Psychol Rev 1993;100(3):366.
25. Bell RH, Biester TW, Tabuenca A, et al. Operative experience of residents in US general surgery programs—a gap between expectation and experience. Ann Surg 2009;249(5):719–24.
26. Chung RS. How much time do residents need to learn operative surgery? Am J Surg 2005;190:351–3.
27. Cooper Z, Meyers M, Keating NL, et al. Resident education and management of end-of-life care: the resident's perspective. J Surg Educ 2010;67(2):79–84.
28. Beckman HB, Frankel RM. The effect of physician behavior on the collection of data. Ann Intern Med 1984;101:692–6.
29. Charon R. Narrative and medicine. N Engl J Med 2004;350(9):862.
30. Dunn GP, Martensen R, Weisssman D, editors. Surgical palliative care—a resident's guide. Essex (CT): Cunniff-Dixon Foundation; 2009. p. 7.
31. Tolstoy L. The death of Ivan Illyich. New York: Bantam Books; 1981.
32. Cassell JA. woman in a surgeon's body. Cambridge (MA): Harvard University Press; 1998.
33. Connolly FK. Walking out on the boys. New York: Farrar, Straus and Giroux; 1998.
34. Thorward J. Unchartered territory. In: The triumph of surgery. New York: Pantheon Books;1960. p. 119. [Richard, Clara Winston, Trans].

Spiritual Dimensions of Surgical Palliative Care

Margaret J. Tarpley, MLS[a],*, John L. Tarpley, MD[b]

KEYWORDS

- Surgeon • Cultural sensitivity • Religion • Spirituality
- Chaplains • End-of-life • Palliative care

"Guérir quelquefois, soulager souvent, consoler toujours" (Cure sometimes, relieve often, comfort always).
> —Ambroise Paré, 16th century surgeon, arguably among the 5 or 6 most important surgeons in medical history.[1]

Pain and suffering are universal human conditions with myriad causes: natural or man-made disasters such as floods or war; lifestyle choices such as smoking or dangerous recreational pursuits; actions such as reckless driving; seemingly random events with catastrophic sequelae such as a person being struck down by a car that failed to yield; emotional upheaval such as relationship difficulties or job loss; and natural disease processes such as cancer or heart problems. Dame Cicely Saunders, founder of the modern hospice movement, used the concept "total pain" to denote the physical, social, emotional, and spiritual components of pain.[2] The career surgeon will likely be required to care for persons with problems that have resulted from all these conditions, and depending on the locale, such as Haiti after the 2010 earthquake, some surgeons might have a lifetime of experience in a much shorter time frame. Surgical procedures have the potential for providing relief from pain and suffering and sometimes even cure. When an operation (if indicated) or nonoperative care offers only temporary respite, the surgeon and the patient and family (or friends) must decide what should be the next step. The primary goal of this article is to encourage surgeons to consider the spiritual dimension of patients and of themselves and to empower surgeons willing to address spiritual considerations.

The authors have nothing to disclose.
The views expressed herein are the author's and do not represent the Department of Veterans Affairs, TVHS.
[a] Department of Surgery, Vanderbilt University, D-4314 MCN, Nashville, TN 37232-2730, USA
[b] Department of Surgery, Vanderbilt University, Veterans Affairs Medical Center, Surgical Service (112), Veterans Affairs Tennessee Valley Healthcare System, Nashville Campus, Nashville, TN 37212, USA
* Corresponding author.
E-mail address: Margaret.tarpley@vanderbilt.edu

The American College of Surgeons (ACS) statement on "Principles Guiding Care at the End of Life," published in 1998 advises: "Respect the dignity of both patients and caregivers; be sensitive to and respectful of the patient's and family's wishes,... recognize, assess, and address psychological, social, and spiritual problems...."[3] Palliative care is recognized globally, with published reports detailing implementation of the principles of palliative care in every continent. The World Health Organization (WHO) defines palliative care as: "an approach that improves the quality of life of patients and their families facing the problem associated with life-threatening illness, through the prevention and relief of suffering by means of early identification and impeccable assessment and treatment of pain and other problems, physical, psycho-social and spiritual.... Palliative care for children is the active total care of the child's body, mind and spirit, and also involves giving support to the family."[4]

Pain and terminal events can affect persons at any age. Both the ACS and WHO acknowledge the spiritual aspects of palliative care for children and adults. However, for relief of physical pain, the low-income countries have far less access to medical narcotics and other analgesics than do the developed countries, such as the United States.[5]

Palliative care services involve skilled professionals who cultivate a relationship with a patient and the patient's family and/or support persons in order to formulate a plan for preventing or relieving suffering, whether it is physical, emotional, or spiritual. The noun *palliation* and the adjective *palliative* noun palliation are derived from the Latin *pallium*, referring to a cloak in ancient Greece and Rome. Pallium evolved into the adjective palliate, meaning cloaked or concealed, and the verb palliate, meaning to cloak, to clothe, or to shelter. In the medical context, palliation currently suggests alleviation of the painful effects of illness, both somatic and spiritual. The need for palliation may arise in any medical context; but the most frequent use of palliative measures and palliative care teams occurs in end-of-life situations, whether from chronic illness, catastrophic events including iatrogenic congenital anomalies, or other situations.[6]

The spiritual dimensions of surgical palliative care encompass recognition of mortality (physician and patient), moral and ethical dilemmas of medical decision making, respect for all belief systems, and responsibility to remain physically and psychologically present. Before initiating a discussion on the spiritual dimensions, the distinctives of palliative care for the surgeon and the surgical team require elucidation, beginning with the dual definitions of the term, the regular involvement with patients who encounter catastrophic events, and the system in which the surgeon operates (See **Box 1**). The first distinctive is that although there may be overlap in medical decision-making thought processes when considering procedures and/or care, the term palliative holds 2 distinct meanings for the surgeon. Surgical palliative procedures are those operations that relate to improving quality of life and/or reducing pain even though unlikely to affect the course of the underlying disease. However, surgical palliative care, also called comfort care, refers to a treatment plan for relief of symptoms and promotion of quality of life for patients under surgical care when no further procedures seem indicated. The decision to perform a palliative procedure is based on the perceived benefit as well as the patient's ability to withstand the operation itself; an example is bypassing a malignant obstruction. When searching the literature via PubMed by linking surgery with palliative care, most of the references actually confuse palliative procedures with noncurative operations. McCahill and colleagues[7] went so far as to declare, "The state of the literature using the word palliation is a mess." When cure is no longer expected, it is essential for the surgeon to explain to the patient/family and the care-giving team that palliative refers primarily to relief of symptoms even though survival may be extended by the intervention.

Box 1
Surgical distinctives of palliative care

Palliative procedures (operations) versus palliative care (comfort)

Disproportionate share of catastrophic event care

Litigation concerns and iatrogenic events

Procedure-driven practice (operations, other procedures, clinics) that limit time for dialogue with patients and families

Reimbursement structures that reward procedures but do not pay for discussions with patients

Shared practice issues; that is, cross-coverage

Outcomes, financial vis-à-vis 30-day survival record, competitiveness in referrals, contracts

Ego, ownership, identity, reputation

American College of Surgeons statement on principles guiding care at the end of life

Moral distress:

    Performing an operative procedure against one's judgment when patient, family, or colleagues insist

    Performing a procedure required for patient transfer guidelines rather than for quality of life

    Surgeon guilt

    Second guessing oneself

    Professional grief when a patient who is under the care of one's resident or colleague or who is a personal friend does poorly or succumbs

---

Accurate communication must always be intentional, and assumptions of understanding must be eliminated. Using the word death may reduce the risk of confusion. Although the exact figures are not available, palliative care services are increasing in numbers locally and globally as the medical community is recognizing the vital service provided by trained palliative care professionals who are fluent in the "language."

A second distinctive of surgical palliative care involves consultation and intervention for patients who have encountered catastrophic events. Although surgeons are not the only physicians who treat survivors of unexpected tragic events, they handle a disproportionate share of these patients. Trauma from a traffic wreck or a burn, a ruptured aortic aneurysm, or an unexpected illness resulting from a fast-acting cancer or an uncontrollable infection, such as necrotizing fasciitis, may adversely affect the adult breadwinner of a family or a child or young adult thought too young to die. The surgeon may face the psychological distress of communicating the bad news of unlikely recovery and then discussing the end-of-life care alternatives with families unprepared for the impending death of someone who, until hours or days ago, was healthy and active. Medical school and residency curricula touch on palliative care, breaking bad news, and communications skills; yet surgeons often feel unprepared and untrained to engage in difficult yet meaningful conversations with patients, families, and colleagues and therefore might choose to request a consultation from a chaplain or the palliative care professional (if one is available).

Third, even when a surgeon recognizes the value of palliative care, the decision to institute such care measures may be complicated by systems-based practice factors such as the assignment of operative mortality, threat of litigation, reaction to iatrogenic events, shared or team coverage because of a trend for a "shift" in the model of coverage, and the finding of time for an honest and meaningful dialogue with the patient and family. The first obstacle is the assignment of responsibility for operative mortality. In the surgical environment, operative mortality is often defined "as the rate of death before hospital discharge or within 30 days after the index procedure."[8] Surgeons are acutely aware of this 30-day window of survival and how it reflects on their own statistics, thus possibly influencing the timing for change of the patient's plan of care. The arbitrary nature of the 30-day standard for operative survival, regardless of the circumstances, is a systems issue and warrants reexamination by policy makers who understand the value of instituting palliative care in a timely manner. "Financial self-interest can become a barrier to palliative caring."[7] Ego investment could be involved as well.

The modern Damoclean sword of litigation, a second obstacle, hangs over the minds of surgeons, especially those who have been personally involved directly or peripherally with a prior law suit; such an obstacle could influence the course of care, even in futile situations. Surgeons are often called upon to place enteral tubes in soon-to-expire patients to facilitate transfer to nursing homes or skilled nursing care centers. Hospital ethics committees, considered essential in accredited medical centers, are relative newcomers in medical administration, with only 1% of the US hospitals having one in 1983. The establishment of ethics committees resulted in part from concerns about possible litigation. In some hospitals, ethics consultations and palliative care consultations can have overlapping territory[9]; but, as a rule, they address different issues. The surgeon who suspects that the patient is unlikely to benefit from further intervention is advised to involve colleagues in the decision process. Seeking an interoperative consultation when continuing or extending the scope of a procedure seems inappropriate provides the surgeon with additional expertise and insulation from self–second-guessing. When a prognosis seems poor preoperatively or postoperatively, the surgeon may request a second opinion in order to validate a change of care plan for himself or herself as well as for the patient and the family or friends. One conundrum with personal implications occurs when change of goals of care (sometimes referred to, inappropriately, as "withdrawal of care") is contemplated when the surgeon feels responsible, rightly or wrongly, for an iatrogenic condition arising from a mishap in the operating room or in the hospital.

Transitioning a surgical care plan from cure to comfort requires dialogue with the patient (if decisional) and with the family or support givers as well as members of the health care team; this is another obstacle. When a surgeon works closely with a group of surgeons who share call on a daily rotation, the sense of personal respon-sibility for an individual patient may be lost unless an intentional effort is made to provide continuity with regular presence and communication. Time constraints of a busy operating room schedule, emergency cases, outpatient clinics, and even teaching responsibilities for those in academic centers restrict the surgeon's opportu-nities for a meaningful conversation necessary to navigate (and negotiate) the path from cure to comfort.

The surgeon's own beliefs, the cultural background and the belief system of the patient and the patient's family, the surgeon-patient interaction, and the role of chap-lains and the pastoral care service are all factors in examining the spiritual dimensions of the process that results in the decision to change the plan of care from treating the disease to providing comfort. When palliative care professionals are consulted, the surgeon may choose to share or even relinquish the decision making to the palliative care team in partnership with the patient and family.

According to several studies the physician's own belief system, whether spiri-tual, religious, or "none," affects medical decision making, consciously and unconsciously.[10–13] In the 1940s, the Vanderbilt chair of surgery, Brooks[14] asserted that in the surgeon-patient relationship the surgeon's interpersonal skills were on par with technical skills, an opinion held by few of his contemporaries. Matthew Walker, chairman of surgery at Meharry Medical College in Nashville, TN, USA, for 39 years, taught that physicians must deal with their own mortality if they were to help patients and families deal with end-of-life decisions.[15] As Woll and colleagues[16] point out: "Patients are not looking to receive direct religious or spiritual care from their surgeons." In a Gallup poll surveying patient thoughts on spirituality and the dying process, respondents desired care givers who listen, discuss fears, and know the patient as a whole person. Hall and Curlin[17] have argued that physician care cannot be neutral regarding religion. They note that secularism is not neutral and that a value-neutral position is not possible and suggest that physicians express their own opinions and emotions. Among his guidelines for religion and spirituality at the end of life, Guinn includes respect for the patient's belief and the admonition to "be sensitive, nonjudgmental, and not proselytizing."[16] Surgeons, all physicians in fact, must guard against boundary violations as addressed by Post and colleagues.[18] Curlin and colleagues[10] noted, "Differences in physicians' religions and spiritual characteristics are associated with differing attitudes and behaviors regarding religion and spirituality in the clinical encounter." Prudence suggests that one wed Socrates' admonition to "know thyself" with the universal "golden rule" of seeking to "treat others as you would wish to be treated," a tenet espoused by virtually all global faith/belief systems.[19]

Hinshaw,[20] a surgeon at the Veterans Affairs Medical Center in Ann Arbor, addressed surgical issues in palliative care and asserted: "Perhaps in no other area of medical specialization does the physician place his/her ego in a more vulnerable position than in the practice of surgery." Outcomes can reflect the surgeon's sense of self-worth. Yet adverse outcomes do occur and "come with the territory." We have all experienced the aphorism: "Hell hath no fury like an internist who has decided it is time to operate." At times, all surgeons are pressed to proceed with operations they are not comfortable with and would prefer not initiating. The presence of pneumatosis, air in the portal venous system, increasing levels of lactate, or even a radiological call of "free air" can often be used to coerce a surgeon to operate when, based on clinical examination and the surgeon's gut instinct, he or she is not certain whether such an operation is to the patient's benefit. Often such procedures are diagnostic rather than therapeutic and nearly always occur in compromised patients with poor physiologic reserve and performance status. The surgeon laments: "I wish I had never operated on that patient!" The surgeon mentally replays the history, physical, investigations, and clinical trajectory of the patient's course over and over again. Instead of deriving joy for trying to provide excellent care and leaving no stone unturned, the surgeon often goes through days of inner debate, self-flagellation, defensiveness, rationalization, justification, regret, loss of emotional energy, and transference of blame. Hopefully, resolution will be found, but the process proves emotionally and often spiritually depleting.

"The tyranny of the lottery shot" can stymie the surgeon, especially in caring for patients with cancer. Quoting the golf putt mantra: "Never up; never in," we at times push the limits of anatomy and physiologic reserve to perform operations of which others, more detached, might later ask: "What was she thinking?" Milch[21] quotes Charles Mayo on the qualities he would want in a surgeon who operates on him as stating: "First he would have to know when to operate, then he would have to know how to operate, then he would have to know when to stop operating." As Art Brooks, Emeritus orthopaedic surgeon at Vanderbilt, instructed his residents: "There is no condition that can't be made worse by an operation." Surgeons expend time, effort, expertise, and energy in seeking to provide skilled, appropriate, timely care. Cases with potential and significant morbidity and real mortality can drain one psychologically, emotionally, and spiritually. One's joy, confidence, and ego can take major hits with the unanticipated or even anticipated adverse outcomes and the requisite remedial work and damage control that ensue. Burnout, depression, and aridity can follow. Surgeons need to be cognizant of their own and their colleagues' stress. An empty tank can lead to depression, overuse of alcohol or drug use, and other risk-taking behaviors. To be able to address the needs of patients and families in the surgical palliative care arena, surgeons and physicians must prioritize their own health and equilibrium. "Physician, heal thyself." Hinshaw[20] notes: "Making time for reflection on the spiritual aspects of one's clinical work is a luxury that seldom is available to busy surgeons." Fatigue, emotional exhaustion, and uncertainty about the meaning and value of one's work can lead to physician burnout. If the possibility of litigation arises, a shared loss transforms to an adversarial relationship.

Moving toward an end-of-life decision of choosing a palliative care plan involves the surgeon and the surgical team, including the nurses, the patient, and the family, in a process that blends scientific, intellectual, social, cultural, and spiritual aspects of the disease process and human relations. Preparing physicians to act in a professional manner and to demonstrate skill in interpersonal relations and communication is required in residency training today. These are 2 of the 6 general "competencies" used to assess the progress of physicians-in-training in all specialties of medicine, not just surgery. The surgeon must interact verbally in an appropriate and hopefully effective manner with the patient and family, even when the surgeon is personally uncomfortable with the topic. Catastrophic events such as motorcycle or all-terrain vehicle crashes with multiple injuries or severe burns involving large areas of the body cause patients to neither appear nor sometimes smell as their families expect. The surgeon and the surgical care team should be aware that family and friends need some warning and preparation about the sight of tubes, drains, bandages, monitors, intravenous fluids, and urine collections or the smells of bodily secretions or chemicals. One difficulty of treating pain and suffering arises when the patient and the family confront the surgeon with the "why" questions. When faced with questions such as "why me" or "what did I do to deserve this," the surgeon who feels unwilling or untrained to attempt answers should involve chaplains or call in the palliative care team when available. These "why" questions are spiritual as well as emotional regardless of the belief system (or lack thereof) of the patient and the patient's support group. Sulmasy[22] stated: "Illness is a spiritual event. Illness grasps persons by the soul and by the body and disturbs them both. Illness ineluctably raises troubling questions of a transcendent nature...about meaning, value, and relationship. These are spiritual questions."

End-of-life situations evoke spiritual concerns that are addressed most comprehensively when the medical care team has some understanding and respect for the patient's belief system, cultural background, and personal identity. The palliative care consultation itself may engender moral distress (a spiritual condition for many) in the physician. "The values that generally underlay goal of care conflicts are the palliative care clinician's values concerning patient comfort, autonomy, quality, and dignity, while the referring clinician is often most concerned about the perceived professional duty to preserve life, along with the emotional impact, ethical propriety, and potential malpractice risk of withholding or withdrawing life sustaining treatments."[23]

Respecting the culture, the beliefs, and the identity of the patient and the patient's family and addressing the spiritual needs is not only the right thing to do but also a task mandated by the Joint Commission, WHO, and numerous medical professional groups. In 1999, Ehmen and colleagues[24] reported that 94% of 177 patients surveyed in an ambulatory care clinic agreed that physicians should ask if patients have beliefs that would influence medical decision making if they became gravely ill. The Joint Commission requires that hospitals address spiritual needs and demonstrate respect for cultural, psychosocial, spiritual, and personal values, beliefs, and preferences as well as gather information relevant to the care, treatment, and services for patients receiving end-of-life care that would include "the social, spiritual, and cultural variables that influence the perceptions and expressions of grief by the patient, family members, or significant others."[25]

Studies demonstrate that quality-of-life indicators in persons with poor prognoses are often higher for those who demonstrate spiritual well-being.[26] Addressing spiritual needs may be achieved in several ways. The intake history queries and physical examination may ask questions regarding religious affiliation, value system, or spiritual beliefs. In the Veterans Affairs Medical Centers, the nursing intake history queries every patient admitted about spiritual or religious beliefs which might affect medical decision making.[15] A formalized and more extensive spiritual history can be elicited with one of the several spiritual assessment tools such as faith, importance and influence, community, address or application (FICA),[27] (spiritual belief system, personal spirituality, integration with a spiritual community, ritualized practices and restrictions, implications for medical care, and terminal events planning (SPIRIT),[28] SpREUK (Germany),[29] and the spiritual distress scale (SDS).[30] Other scales are being studied for specific cultures such as Native Americans[31] or for geographic areas such as Korea.[32] The ideal time for asking the simple questions or administering these assessment tools would be before deterioration or admission, on admission, or early in the hospital course when the patient and family are able to interact thoughtfully without the stress of impending demise.

Knowing if a patient and the family are religious in the sense of adhering to an organized belief system, are spiritual in the sense of acknowledging some higher power of the supernatural or natural world, or find life meaning in work or recreation will give the health care team knowledge to better meet their needs if deterioration in the physical condition occurs. When religion defines who a person is, such as a Jehovah's Witness, an evangelical Christian, or an Orthodox Jew, religious beliefs will certainly influence medical decisions. Communication is essential in order to find out what is acceptable and if religious or community leaders should be called in for consultation and support. Balboni and colleagues,[33] addressing patients with advanced cancer, noted that 88% of those queried attested that religion was at least somewhat important. About 47% noted that their spiritual needs were either minimally supported or not supported by their own religious community, whereas 72% noted that their spiritual needs were either minimally supported or not supported by the medical systems. Ferrell[34] editorialized that this was "a seriously unmet need in the vast majority of (cancer) patients in our care." She advocated that oncologists needed to master the skills of taking a basic assessment of spiritual needs, assess themselves, and become advocates for the chaplaincy. In a most useful contribution, Lo and colleagues[35] offered "a practical guide for physicians." They presented phrases to help elicit the patient's concerns; they described pitfalls in discussions about spiritual and religious issues near the end of life and provided goals for physicians when discussing spiritual and religious issues with patients and families near the end of life.[35] An important task of a medical professional, the surgeon, the chaplain, the palliative care physician, or the nurse, is simply talking to the patient or, if the patient cannot communicate, talking to the family members.

Allowing the patient and/or family to ask questions or share their stories of the patient can be therapeutic for everyone involved.

Whether traditions and taboos are religious, cultural, or social, respecting and tolerating them can be critical for persons such as followers of African religions that do not permit amputations or stomas for palliation or even cure or Jehovah's Witnesses who will tolerate no blood products. Followers of Hinduism shun autopsies not required by law.[36] In the Islamic culture, the deceased person's head should face toward Mecca and the body should be bathed by the family immediately after death.[37] Rites and ceremonies may be crucial to the healing process, even when cure will not occur. Creative accommodation to practices such as prayer or candles (battery-powered) or even sacrificing a chicken (parking lot or hospital kitchen) may send the nonverbal message of acceptance and respect. Dietary restrictions should be honored. Demands for (or refusal of) medical caregivers of a specific gender should be given consideration even if inconvenient when it is possible to accede to these requests or should be gently explained if it is impossible to arrange. Honesty should be maintained without removing all hope[38] but ethnocentricity in communication should be eschewed and words should be chosen with care. "The western 'right to know' can be in direct conflict with the perceived power of the spoken word; what is not said explicitly may not become reality" for peoples in some non-western cultures.[20] In a local or international environment, cultural humility and empathy are essential.[39] The gay, lesbian, bisexual, and transgender communities present complex health care needs deserving of quality care and respect. One study showed stronger support in the gay community for palliative care and completion of advanced directives than in the adult population at large.[40] However, domestic partners in same-sex relationships may not have the same legal rights to participate in end-of-life decision making[41] as those whose family structures are more "traditional."

Addressing the spiritual needs of patients may best be accomplished by requesting a chaplain consult or asking the patient and /or family who they want to involve, such as their rabbi, imam, priest, or pastor. For the nonreligious or nonspiritual or for those involved in legal restrictions, such as those faced by same-sex partners, a social worker may provide emotional or social support. The palliative care professionals and chaplains are knowledgeable in emotional, social, and spiritual support.

When palliative measures or comfort care (sometimes called "withdrawal of care," a phrase that may, unfortunately, be misinterpreted to mean all care) are under consideration by the patient and the family involved as well as the surgical team, chaplains and the pastoral care team offer trained support to those persons dealing with impending death regardless of faith systems or lack thereof. Chaplains are often underutilized by physicians as well as surgeons. Studies show that nurses are more likely than physicians to request a chaplain consult.[42,43] Because of their specialized training to counsel persons in time of uncertainty, suffering, and the possibility of poor outcomes (including death), chaplains should be invited to participate in rounds and be introduced to patients and families and hospital staff who may require their assistance and ministry. At Vanderbilt University Medical Center in Nashville, the chaplains are on call with the trauma team whenever the team must communicate adverse events or other bad news.

"Listening is one of the greatest spiritual gifts a chaplain [or a surgeon] can give a suffering patient."[20] Chaplains, like the palliative care teams, may well have more time than surgeons to spend talking with patients and families. The surgeons, nurses, and other health care professionals may also require the ministry of chaplains. Certified hospital chaplains have graduate theological education as well as 1600 hours of supervised training and are competent to help the patient and family understand the issues involved and opt for comfort care when their decisions might be complicated by the publicity given to accounts such as the Terry Schiavo case and controversies surrounding euthanasia.

Along with chaplains, the palliative care physicians have a year of fellowship. Fellowship training for palliative medicine physicians includes experience in responding to the difficult questions that arise as a change of care plan is contemplated; they have dual abilities when talking to patients, responding to the angst and emotional pain that frequently accompanies the "why" questions and then, to develop a treatment plan that allows pain and suffering issues to be addressed medically as well as psychologically.

The wise use of scarce health care resources is considered by most to be an ethical, moral, and even a spiritual issue. While relief of pain and suffering remains the primary goal of palliative care, evidence exists that palliative care is also cost-effective and decreases daily costs in hospital as well as overall costs for a terminal event.[44,45]

In this era of evidence-based medicine, it must be proved that palliative care (not necessarily surgical) has significant effect on quality of life and satisfaction with care. Zimmerman and colleagues[46] performed such a review of randomized controlled trials and judged that only 22 of 396 met their criteria and showed some evidence for effectiveness of family satisfaction, improved quality of life, and cost benefits. Further study with carefully planned trials was recommended.

After this dissertation on the spiritual dimensions of surgical palliative care with the focus on patient, family, surgeon, nurse, chaplain, palliative care professional, and the system within which all of these persons interact expressing their own beliefs, culture, ethics, gender, and educational opportunities, the authors offer a brief list of practical recommendations:

1. Be aware of your own worldview or "lens" as you assist patients and families make medical or end-of-life decisions.
2. Make certain that the spiritual needs of the patient and the family/support persons are addressed even if they cannot be met.
3. As the likelihood of improvement disappears, be present and be available. Do not abandon the patient and family when medical solutions are no longer options.
4. Maintain honesty without removing all hope.
5. Use the pastoral care and social work services early rather than late. Include the chaplains on rounds.
6. Call in the palliative care professional when one is available.
7. Healing and cure are not synonymous.

ACKNOWLEDGMENTS

Dr Mohana Karlekar, Director, Vanderbilt University Palliative Care, provided an experienced viewpoint as well as references and advice. Dr Karlekar and Dr Kyla Terhune, Chief Resident in General Surgery, offered invaluable insights into the surgeon-patient-family interaction.

REFERENCES

1. Standards of conduct: it's the right thing to do. Available at: http://www.studergroup. com/newsletter/Vol1_Issue4/vol1_i4_sec8.htm. Accessed September 28, 2010.
2. Krouse RS, Jonasson O, Milch RA, et al. An evolving strategy for surgical care. J Am Coll Surg 2004;198:149–55.

3. Statements of the college. [ST-28] Principles guiding care at the end of life. Available at: http://www.facs.org/fellows_info/statements/st-28.html. Accessed September 28, 2010.
4. World Health Organization. WHO definition of palliative care. Available at: http://www.who.int/cancer/palliative/definition/en/. Accessed September 8, 2010.
5. McNeil DG Jr. Drugs banned, many of world's poor suffer in pain. 2007. Available at: http://www.nytimes.com/2007/09/10/health/10pain.html?_r=1&th=&adxnnl=1&oref=slogin&emc=th&adxnnlx=1189425627-zbx8wT3JR6mrUvkZZyLOPQ. Accessed September 28, 2010.
6. MedicineNet.com. Definition of palliation. Available at: http://www.medterms.com/script/main/art.asp?articlekey=9048. Accessed September 30, 2010.
7. McCahill LE, Dunn GP, Mosenthal AC, et al. Palliation as a core surgical principle: part 1. J Am Coll Surg 2004;199:149–60.
8. Birkmeyer JD, Siewers AE, Finlayson EV, et al. Hospital volume and surgical mortality in the United States. N Engl J Med 2002;346(15):1128–37.
9. Aulisio MP, Arnold RM. Role of the ethics committee: helping to address value conflicts or uncertainties. Chest 2008;134(2):417–24.
10. Curlin FA, Chin MH, Sellergren SA, et al. The association of physicians' religious characteristics with their attitudes and self-reported behaviors regarding religion and spirituality in the clinical encounter. Med Care 2006;44:446–53.
11. Curlin FA, Sellergren SA, Lantos JD, et al. Physicians' observations and interpretations of the influence of religion and spirituality on health. Arch Intern Med 2007; 167:649–54.
12. Barr P. Relationship of neonatologists' end-of-life decisions to their personal fear of death. Arch Dis Child Fetal Neonatal Ed 2007;92(2):F104–7.
13. Catlin EA, Cadge W, Ecklund EH, et al. The spiritual and religious identities, beliefs, and practices of academic pediatricians in the United States. Acad Med 2008;83:1146–52.
14. Brooks B. Address of the President: psychosomatic surgery. Ann Surg 1944;119: 289–99.
15. Tarpley JL, Tarpley MJ. Spirituality in surgical practice. J Am Coll Surg 2002;194: 642–7.
16. Woll ML, Hinshaw DB, Pawlik TM. Spirituality and religion in the care of surgical oncology patients with life-threatening or advanced illnesses. Ann Surg Oncol 2008;15:3048–57.
17. Hall DE, Curlin F. Can physicians' care be neutral regarding religion? Acad Med 2004;79:677–9.
18. Post SG, Puchalski CM, Larson DB. Physicians and patient spirituality: professional boundaries, competency, and ethics. Ann Intern Med 2000;132:578–83.
19. Milan J, McKenna P. Golden rule workshop guidelines 2002. Available at: http://www.pflaum.com/goldrule/guideline.htm. Accessed September 25, 2010.
20. Hinshaw DB. Spiritual issues in surgical palliative care. Surg Clin North Am 2005; 85:257–72.
21. Milch RA. Surgical palliative care. Semin Oncol 2005;32:165–8.
22. Sulmasy DP. Is medicine a spiritual practice? Acad Med 1999;74:1002–5.
23. Weissman DE. Palliative care in moral distress. J Palliat Med 2009;12:865–6.
24. Ehman JW, Ott BB, Short TH, et al. Do patients want physicians to inquire about their spiritual or religious beliefs if they become gravely ill? Arch Intern Med 1999; 159:1803–6.
25. The Joint Commission. Comprehensive Accreditation Manual for Hospitals: The Official Handbook (CAMH). Oakbrook Terrace (IL): Joint Commission Resources; 2008.

26. Harris BA, Berger AM, Mitchell SA, et al. Spiritual well-being in long-term survivors with chronic graft-versus-host disease after hematopoietic stem cell transplantation. J Support Oncol 2010;8:119–25.
27. Borneman T, Ferrell B, Puchalski CM. Evaluation of the FICA tool for spiritual assessment. J Pain Symptom Manage 2010;40:163–73.
28. Maugans TA. The SPIRITual history. Arch Fam Med 1996;5:11–6.
29. Bussing A. The SpREUK-SF10 questionnaire as a rapid measure of spiritual search and religious trust in patients with chronic diseases. Zhong Xi Yi Jie He Xue Bao 2010;8:832–41.
30. Ku YL, Kuo SM, Yao CY. Establishing the validity of a spiritual distress scale for cancer patients hospitalized in southern Taiwan. Int J Palliat Nurs 2010;16:134–8.
31. Hodge DR, Limb GE. A Native American perspective on spiritual assessment: the strengths and limitations of a complementary set of assessment tools. Health Soc Work 2010;35:121–31.
32. Yong J, Kim J, Han SS, et al. Development and validation of a scale assessing spiritual needs for Korean patients with cancer. J Palliat Care 2008;24:240–6.
33. Balboni TA, Vanderwerker LC, Block SD, et al. Religiousness and spiritual support among advanced cancer patients and associations with end-of-life treatment preferences and quality of life. J Clin Oncol 2007;25:555–60.
34. Ferrell B. Meeting spiritual needs: what is an oncologist to do? J Clin Oncol 2007;25:467–8.
35. Lo B, Ruston D, Kates LW, et al. Working group on religious and spiritual issues at the end of life. Discussing religious and spiritual issues at the end of life: a practical guide for physicians. JAMA 2002;287:749–54.
36. Sulmasy DP. Spirituality, religion, and clinical care. Chest 2009;135:1634–42.
37. Sarhill N, LeGrand S, Islambouli R, et al. The terminally ill Muslim: death and dying from the Muslim perspective. Am J Hosp Palliat Care 2001;18:251–5.
38. McCahill LE, Krouse RS, Chu DZ, et al. Decision making in palliative surgery. J Am Coll Surg 2002;195:411–22.
39. Paice JA, Ferrell B, Coyle N, et al. Living and dying in East Africa: implementing the End-of-Life Nursing Education Consortium curriculum in Tanzania. Clin J Oncol Nurs 2010;14:161–6.
40. Stein GL, Bonuck KA. Attitudes on end-of-life care and advance. J Palliat Med 2001;4:173–90.
41. Smolinski KM, Colón Y. Silent voices and invisible walls: exploring end of life care with lesbians and gay men. J Psychosoc Oncol 2006;24:51–64.
42. Vanderwerker LC, Flannelly KJ, Galek K, et al. What do chaplains really do? III. Referrals in the New York Chaplaincy Study. J Health Care Chaplain 2008;14:57–73.
43. Flannelly KJ, Weaver AJ, Handzo GF. A three-year study of chaplains' professional activities at Memorial Sloan-Kettering Cancer Center in New York City. Psychooncology 2003;12:760–8.
44. Smith TJ, Cassel JB. Cost and non-clinical outcomes of palliative care. J Pain Symptom Manage 2009;38:32–44.
45. Penrod JD, Deb P, Dellenbaugh C, et al. Hospital-based palliative care consultation: effects on hospital cost. J Palliat Med 2010;13:973–9.
46. Zimmermann C, Riechelmann R, Krzyzanowska M, et al. Effectiveness of specialized palliative care: a systematic review. JAMA 2008;299:1698–709.

Inpatient Palliative Care Consultation: Enhancing Quality of Care for Surgical Patients by Collaboration

Michael D. Adolph, MD

KEYWORDS

• Palliative care • Surgery • Consultation • Quality • Satisfaction

With 1300 hospitals claiming to have a palliative care program, and nearly 90 palliative care fellowships poised to graduate hundreds of trainees each year, the hospital-based surgeon will likely encounter palliative care services more frequently.[1] This article proposes that the surgeon can use inpatient palliative care services in four broad clinical settings to benefit their patients. In addition, palliative care services with assumptions about surgical patient care may benefit, from a learning perspective, by collaborating with surgical colleagues to improve care for mutual patients. After all, only a small number of physicians who are board certified in palliative care are surgeons.

Because the palliative care field is undergoing exponential growth, setting expectations and anticipating occasional misunderstandings are important measures as an organization embraces palliative care consultations. As the course of a patient's clinical trajectory crosses the path of both a surgeon and a palliative care clinician, potential areas of conflict may arise, but collaboration can prevail over conflict. Finally, this article examines options for system changes, because surgeons may identify a broader need to include palliative care principles beyond consultation services, as other organizations and nations have discovered.

Surgeons may consult with palliative care colleagues to help patients and families manage symptoms, cope with the distress of acute and chronic illness, manage complex decisions at end-of-life, and negotiate through a critical illness (or combinations thereof). These clinical areas are clearly expansive; in fact the National Quality

The author has no relevant industrial or financial relationships to disclose.

Division of Surgical Oncology, Pain & Palliative Medicine Service, Center for Palliative Care, James Cancer Hospital and Solove Research Institute, Ohio State University College of Medicine, 453 West 10th Avenue, Atwell Hall 246, Columbus, OH 43210, USA

E-mail address: michael.adolph@osumc.edu

Surg Clin N Am 91 (2011) 317–324
doi:10.1016/j.suc.2010.12.002
0039-6109/11/$ – see front matter © 2011 Elsevier Inc. All rights reserved.

Forum recently reviewed 38 preferred practices for hospice and palliative care.[2] They found it reasonable to promote eight domains of palliative care (**Box 1**) in their *Clinical Practice Guidelines for Quality Palliative Care* to simplify evidenced-based practice for the palliative care field.[3] Palliative care physicians base their practice on a comprehensive assessment from each of these domains. Therefore, surgeons who prefer more

---

Box 1
Domains of palliative care and examples of interventions

Domain 1: Structure and processes of care

Education and support to patient, family, and health care staff

Family conference to review care plan; a primary procedure for a palliative care specialist

Discharge planning and coordination with primary service and social work

Domain 2: Physical aspects of care

Pharmacologic pain management

Nonpharmacologic pain management

Nonpain symptom management

Domain 3: Psychological and psychiatric aspects of care

Enhancing adjustment and coping with distress for patients and family

Diagnosing and treating anxiety or depression

Identifying anticipatory grief in patient and family

Domain 4: Social aspects of care

Developing and implementing a comprehensive social care plan to address the social and practical needs of patients and caregivers

Family conference to discuss goals of care

Domain 5: Spiritual, religious, and existential aspects of care

Identifying meaning and purpose from the patient's perspective

Identifying a patient's specific spiritual practices and providing direction to resources and personnel to meet these needs in the context of illness

Domain 6: Cultural Aspects of Care

Incorporating cultural assessment as a component of comprehensive palliative care to identify areas such as communication needs or locus of decision-making

Domain 7: Care of the imminently dying patient

Decision-making regarding initiation of life-prolonging treatment

Assisting with withdrawal of life support in medical futility cases

Hospice referral

Domain 8: Ethical and legal aspects of care

Decisional capacity assessment

Clarifying code status

Assisting with advance directives

Adapted from National Consensus Project for Quality PalliativeCare. Clinical practice guidelines for quality palliative care. 2nd edition. Available at: http://www.nationalconsensusproject.org. Accessed August 2, 2010; with permission.

limited interventions should specify this to clarify expectations. Requests for consultation should be explicit and ideally communicated verbally with palliative care colleagues so that no presumptions are made by either the surgical or palliative care team. These dynamic clinical situations are often emotionally charged and already burdensome for patients and families, and therefore unified and clear clinical collaboration with palliative care colleagues is extremely important.

Aside from expectations, another source of potential conflict between surgeons and palliative care colleagues may involve discordant practice perspectives. Patients in a surgeon's population rarely die, but the palliative care clinicians' patients rarely live a lengthy time. The patients seen by surgeons who seem most likely to die are generally rescued through surgical intervention, critical care support, or both. Therefore, surgeons may have difficulty recognizing death; palliative care colleagues may have difficulty becoming comfortable with patients living with chronic surgical illness.

If surgeons do not want help with end-of-life care at a specific juncture in a patient's trajectory, those intentions should be made clear to the palliative care colleagues. Alternatively, surgeons can at least communicate to their palliative care colleagues at what point they would propose opening discussions about end-of-life issues. Surgeons should make their intentions clear, because they are trained to contemplate surgical considerations that are second nature to them, but which are often outside the training and experience of most palliative care clinicians.

End-of-life care is entrenched in palliative care practice[2] and fellowship training.[4] If end-of-life care is the prevailing tool possessed by palliative care colleagues in a surgeon's facility, then the entire world may seem a nail for them to apply this dominant hammer: comprehensive end-of-life care. However, although end-of-life care is a part of palliative care, it is surely not all of palliative care. The practice and training of palliative care colleagues may involve disease management support for chronic surgical illnesses. Emerging opinions of national consensus organizations are clear: that palliative care needs of patients and families begin at diagnosis. For example, the American Society for Clinical Oncology (ASCO) states that interdisciplinary palliative care should begin at initial diagnosis of cancer.[5] Moreover, recent innovations in the field of ambulatory palliative care have yet to diffuse throughout the palliative care world.[6] Depending on the nature of their training and practice, palliative care clinicians and trainees may have limited experience in a setting of ambulatory care and chronic disease management, which may seem second nature to surgeons.

However, surgeons should also be aware that their close relationship with their patients may be a principal barrier to accurate prognostication of a patient's imminent death. Prognosticating is stressful for all,[7] and clinicians with a limited time in a clinical relationship have been shown to prognosticate better than those who have an established, lengthy patient–doctor relationship.[8] Some investigators propose that the intimacy exemplified by the surgeon's hands inside a patient, and the resulting surgeon–patient relationship, create a level of "buy-in" that makes delivering adverse prognoses and withdrawing care for an individual patient very difficult decision-making processes for surgeons. In a qualitative study, Schwarze and colleagues[9] interviewed 10 surgeons and found that surgical buy-in begins in the preoperative period and is grounded in a surgeon's sense of responsibility for surgical outcomes; this preoperative buy-in can influence decision-making as a patient's clinical trajectory unfolds, particularly when adverse clinical events arise.

Based on literature in their specialty journals, palliative care clinicians are likely to enter a clinical situation presuming inadequate pain control,[10] excessive patient and family distress,[11] or inadequately addressed prognostic expectations or communications.[12,13] These assumptions should not be surprising to the surgical world; surgeons do not routinely obtain this kind of training in surgical residency curricula.[1] The skillful and adept palliative care colleague should collaborate and present thoughtful recommendations with the intent to form long-term relationships with their surgical colleagues and provide surgical patients with access to interdisciplinary palliative care.

HELPING PATIENTS AND FAMILIES MANAGE SYMPTOMS AND COPE WITH DISTRESS OF ACUTE OR CHRONIC ILLNESS

Patients with advanced age, multiple comorbidities,[14] complicated disease, or surgical complications are more likely to experience reoperation, prolonged hospitalization, inpatient readmissions, or frequent access to postoperative ambulatory care.[15] According to data from the National Surgical Quality Improvement Program, the 10 most commonly performed general surgery procedures account for more than 60% of complications.[16] In vascular surgery, the 4 most commonly performed procedures account for more than 75% of complications.[17] These patients are at higher risk for symptoms and distress from acute and chronic surgical illness. Palliative medicine physicians are trained to be experts in symptom management,[18] including cancer pain, acute and chronic pain, and symptoms related to advanced and terminal illness.[2] For patients experiencing persistent symptoms despite addressing or excluding surgically reversible problems, palliative care clinicians are an available resource for collaboration to medically manage symptoms, including symptom clusters.[19,20]

Patients and families experiencing the distress of acute or chronic surgical illness can obtain relief through accessing interdisciplinary palliative care resources. Improved patient satisfaction and communication from all caregivers was perceived by 1517 patients surveyed in an evaluation of inpatient palliative care services in San Francisco, Denver, and Portland.[21] An inpatient palliative care consult may also be the point of care to access ambulatory palliative care services. Temel and colleagues[6] randomized 151 patients with metastatic lung cancer to early palliative care versus usual care shortly after diagnosis. Patients receiving early palliative care averaged four clinic visits (highest was eight visits) over the next 12 weeks. Study patients had statistically significant improvements in quality of life compared with controls, as assessed using three scales. Notably, survival for the study group exceeded that of the control group (mean, 11.6 months; 95% CI, 6.4–16.9 months vs mean, 8.9 months; 95% CI, 6.3–11.4 months).

For surgical oncology patients, palliative care and best supportive care are not categorically synonymous; in fact, best supportive care, as given in usual care arms of cancer clinical trials, has methodological deficits and possibly ethical problems as currently applied in the scientific literature.[22] It may be likely that surgical oncologists will enhance the quality of surgical patient care more with a palliative care consultation than with an institution's practice of best supportive care.

HELPING PATIENTS AND FAMILIES MANAGE COMPLEX DECISIONS AT END-OF-LIFE

As the trajectory of an illness involves functional decline or impending death, conscious patients and their families shift their goals to what matters most to them,[23] including the need to prepare.[24] Moreover, what becomes important to patients may be discordant with what physicians perceive as important at the end of life.[12] Palliative care colleagues can help surgeons and their patients clarify goals and manage uncertainty by supporting patients and families in the days, weeks, and months at or near the end of life. Inpatient palliative care consultation has been shown to improve satisfaction of patients, families, and referring clinicians.[25–27]

HELPING PATIENTS AND FAMILIES NEGOTIATE THROUGH A CRITICAL ILLNESS

Modern technological advances and the uncertainty of advanced illness have caused a greater recognition of the challenges of surgical critical care, namely how to balance a responsibility to rescue vulnerable survivors, yet fulfill the obligation to comfort patients and families. Even when critical care works well, it is burdensome for all patients and families.[28,29] These stakeholder tensions have led to a paradigm shift away from delaying palliative care until a patient is nearly dead, to integrating palliative care principles a priori for all admissions to the intensive care unit (ICU).[30,31] Intensivists and palliative care colleagues should develop skill and expertise in developing care plans to meet the specific needs of patients and families encountering critical illness, because the needs for surgically critically ill patients are unique.[32]

The ICU is a hazardous place for the mental health of all who enter. Family members of patients in the ICU show increased rates of depression and may show symptoms similar to posttraumatic stress disorder (PTSD) if their loved one dies in the ICU.[33,34] Nurses in the ICU are also at risk for PTSD-like symptoms.[35] A study of 5268 clinicians in 323 ICUs in 24 countries showed that 71% of physicians and nurses surveyed have encountered workplace conflict associated with substantial job strain. To address this emotionally toxic environment, the American College of Critical Care Medicine produced guidelines for implementing better support of family in the patient-centered ICU.[36] Systems change in the ICU may be the best approach to mitigate these environmental hazards.

QUALITY IMPROVEMENT AND SYSTEMS CHANGE APPROACHES

Once the practicing surgeon has encountered and embraced palliative care principles and collaborations into their practice, patterns of care and barriers to palliative care will become evident. Transforming a team,[37] an organization,[38] or a nation[39] to implement better palliative care may involve starting a quality improvement project in surgical practices. For example, the author's palliative medicine service collaborated daily with their thoracic surgical oncology service to implement processes to improve pain control and other outcomes. Through implementing a case-based education approach, the services shared information on each specific patient and saw sustained improvements in satisfaction with pain management among patients with lung cancer, which persisted even after the daily collaboration ceased.[37] During the same period, the authors' series of more than 528 surgical inpatients showed that risk-adjusted length of stay improved, costs decreased, and numbers of patients enrolled in thoracic oncology cancer therapy trials increased by 35%.

Even the palliative care community has recognized the gap between guideline recommendations and their implementation for improving delivery of palliative care.[29] The Center for the Advancement of Palliative Care, in conjunction with many national leaders in surgical critical care, have endorsed a team-based stakeholder approach to improve critical palliative care through well-structured intensive care unit palliative care initiatives.[29] The principles outlined in their detailed approach, including Web-based resources for this National Institutes of Health–funded endeavor, provide a useful template for clinical quality improvement in any setting.[40]

SUMMARY

Surgeons may select from a broad range of services provided by palliative care teams in their hospital. The rationale for a palliative care consultation request should be explicit to avoid presumptions made by either the surgical or palliative care team.

Inpatient palliative care consultation has been shown to improve quality of care, including quality of life and satisfaction of patients, families, and referring clinicians. Surgeons can play an important role in expanding access and quality of care for surgical patients in need of interdisciplinary palliative care services through collaborating with palliative care service colleagues in their hospital.

REFERENCES

1. Adolph MD, Dunn GP. Postgraduate palliative medicine training for the surgeon: an update on ABMS subspecialty certification. Bull Am Coll Surg 2009;94(2):6–13 47.
2. National Consensus Project for Quality PalliativeCare. Clinical practice guidelines for quality palliative care, 2nd edition. Available at: http://www.nationalconsensusproject.org/Guidelines_Download.asp. Accessed August 2, 2010.
3. Ferrell B, Connor SR, Cordes A, et al. The national agenda for quality palliative care: the National Consensus Project and the National Quality Forum. J Pain Symptom Manage 2007;33(6):737–44.
4. Acgme. Hospice and palliative medicine core competencies. 2007. Available at: http://www.acgme.org/outcome/implement/HPM_Competencies_Ver_2_1.pdf. Accessed July 21, 2010.
5. Ferris FD, Bruera E, Cherny N, et al. palliative cancer care a decade later: accomplishments, the need, next steps–from the American Society of Clinical Oncology. J Clin Oncol 2009;27(18):3052–8.
6. Temel JS, Greer JA, Muzikansky A, et al. Early palliative care for patients with metastatic non-small-cell lung cancer. N Engl J Med 2010;363(8):733–42.
7. Christakis NA, Iwashyna TJ. Attitude and self-reported practice regarding prognostication in a national sample of internists. Arch Intern Med 1998;158(21):2389–95.
8. Christakis NA, Lamont EB. Extent and determinants of error in physicians' prognoses in terminally ill patients: prospective cohort study. West J Med 2000;172(5):310–3.
9. Schwarze ML, Bradley CT, Brasel KJ. Surgical "buy-in": the contractual relationship between surgeons and patients that influences decisions regarding life-supporting therapy. Crit Care Med 2010;38(3):843–8.
10. The SUPPORT Principal Investigators. A controlled trial to improve care for seriously ill hospitalized patients. The study to understand prognoses and preferences for outcomes and risks of treatments (SUPPORT). JAMA 1995;274(20):1591–8 [Erratum: JAMA 1996;24;275(16):1232].
11. Yates P, Aranda S, Edwards H, et al. Family caregivers' experiences and involvement with cancer pain management. J Palliat Care 2004;20(4):287–96.
12. Steinhauser KE, Christakis NA, Clipp EC, et al. Factors considered important at the end of life by patients, family, physicians, and other care providers. JAMA 2000;284(19):2476–82.
13. Bradley CT, Brasel KJ. Core competencies in palliative care for surgeons: interpersonal and communication skills. Am J Hosp Palliat Care 2007;24(6):499–507.
14. Merkow RP, Bilimoria KY, Cohen ME, et al. Variability in reoperation rates at 182 hospitals: a potential target for quality improvement. J Am Coll Surg 2009;209(5):557–64.
15. Bilimoria KY, Cohen ME, Ingraham AM, et al. Effect of postdischarge morbidity and mortality on comparisons of hospital surgical quality. Ann Surg 2010;252(1):183–90.

16. Schilling PL, Dimick JB, Birkmeyer JD. Prioritizing quality improvement in general surgery. J Am Coll Surg 2008;207(5):698–704.
17. Schilling PL, Dimick JB, Birkmeyer JD. Prioritizing quality improvement in vascular surgery. Surg Innov 2010;17(2):127–31.
18. von Gunten C, Buckholz G, Ferris FD. Education and training in palliative medicine: training specialists in palliative medicine. In: Hanks GW, Cherny NI, Christatkis NA, editors. Oxford textbook of palliative medicine. 4th edition. Oxford (UK): Oxford University Press; 2010. p. 1586–96.
19. Paice JA. Assessment of symptom clusters in people with cancer. J Natl Cancer Inst Monogr 2004;32:98–102.
20. Ciemins EL, Blum L, Nunley M, et al. The economic and clinical impact of an inpatient palliative care consultation service: a multifaceted approach. J Palliat Med 2007;10(6):1347–55.
21. Gade G, Venohr I, Conner D, et al. Impact of an inpatient palliative care team: a randomized control trial. J Palliat Med 2008;11(2):180–90.
22. Cherny NI, Abernethy AP, Strasser F, et al. Improving the methodologic and ethical validity of best supportive care studies in oncology: lessons from a systematic review. J Clin Oncol 2009;27(32):5476–86.
23. Heyland DK, Dodek P, Rocker G, et al. What matters most in end-of-life care: perceptions of seriously ill patients and their family members. CMAJ 2006; 174(5):627–33.
24. Aspinal F, Hughes R, Dunckley M, et al. What is important to measure in the last months and weeks of life?: A modified nominal group study. Int J Nurs Stud 2006; 43(4):393–403.
25. Bookbinder M, Coyle N, Kiss M, et al. Implementing national standards for cancer pain management: program model and evaluation. J Pain Symptom Manage 1996;12(6):334–47.
26. O'Mahony S, Blank A, Zallman L, et al. The benefits of a hospital-based inpatient palliative care consultation service: Preliminary outcome data. J Palliat Med 2005; 8(5):1033–9.
27. Manfredi PL, Morrison RS, Morris J, et al. Palliative care consultations: how do they impact the care of hospitalized patients? J Pain Symptom Manage 2000; 20(3):166–73.
28. Nelson JE, Puntillo KA, Pronovost PJ, et al. In their own words: patients and families define high-quality palliative care in the intensive care unit. Crit Care Med 2010;38(3):808–18.
29. Nelson JE, Bassett R, Boss RD, et al. Models for structuring a clinical initiative to enhance palliative care in the intensive care unit: a report from the IPAL-ICU Project (Improving Palliative Care in the ICU). Crit Care Med 2010;38(9): 1765–72.
30. Mosenthal A, Murphy P. Interdisciplinary model for palliative care in the trauma and surgical intensive care unit: Robert Wood Johnson Foundation Demonstration Project for Improving Palliative Care in the Intensive Care Unit. Crit Care Med 2006;34(11):S399.
31. Mosenthal A, Murphy P, Barker L, et al. Changing the culture around end-of-life care in the trauma intensive care unit. J Trauma 2008;64(6):1587.
32. Bradley C, Weaver J, Brasel K. Addressing access to palliative care services in the surgical intensive care unit. Surgery 2010;147(6):871–7.
33. Siegel MD, Hayes E, Vanderwerker LC, et al. Psychiatric illness in the next of kin of patients who die in the intensive care unit. Crit Care Med 2008;36(6): 1722–8.

34. Azoulay E, Pochard F, Kentish-Barnes N, et al. Risk of post-traumatic stress symptoms in family members of intensive care unit patients. Am J Respir Crit Care Med 2005;171(9):987–94.
35. Mealer M, Shelton A, Berg B, et al. Increased prevalence of post traumatic stress disorder symptoms in critical care nurses. Am J Respir Crit Care Med 2007; 175(7):693–7.
36. Armstrong D, Davidson J, Powers K, et al. Clinical practice guidelines for support of the family in the patient-centered intensive care unit: American College of Critical Care Medicine Task Force 2004–2005. Crit Care Med 2007;35(2):605.
37. Adolph MD, Taylor RM, Ross PM, et al. Evaluating cancer patient satisfaction before and after daily multidisciplinary care for thoracic surgery inpatients. J Clin Oncol 2009;27(18S):9605.
38. Bookbinder M, Blank AE, Arney E, et al. Improving end-of-life care: development and pilot-test of a clinical pathway. J Pain Symptom Manage 2005;29(6):529–43.
39. Ellershaw JE, Murphy D. The Liverpool Care Pathway (LCP) influencing the UK national agenda on care of the dying. Int J Palliat Nurs 2005;11(3):132–4.
40. Center for the Advancement of Palliative Care. Improving palliative care in the ICU- the IPAL-ICU project. 2010. Available at: http://www.capc.org/ipal-icu/. Accessed August 21, 2010.

Palliative Medicine in the Surgical Intensive Care Unit and Trauma

Christine C. Toevs, MD, FCCM

KEYWORDS

• Palliative care • Trauma • Surgical intensive care unit
• End of life • Family support • Communication

Palliative Medicine is a new discipline that focuses on all aspects of a person in relation to medicine: physical, spiritual, and emotional. The purpose of palliative medicine is to prevent and relieve suffering and to help patients and their families set informed goals of care and treatment. Palliative medicine can be provided along with life-prolonging treatment or as the main focus of treatment.

The intensive care unit (ICU) plays a prominent role in medical care in the United States today. National data suggest 30% to 40% of all patients admitted to the ICU will die while in the ICU or before hospital discharge, and 22% of all deaths in the United States now occur in or after admission to an ICU. Palliative medicine has an increasing role and presence in the ICU. The purpose of this article is to discuss the growing and essential role of palliative medicine to comprehensive patient-centered care in the surgical intensive care unit (SICU) and trauma.

LONG-TERM OUTCOMES IN SICU AND TRAUMA

In the past several years, studies have begun to address the long-term outcomes of patients following ICU admission. Wunsch and colleagues[1] looked at 35,308 Medicare ICU subjects who survived to hospital discharge. They noted that ICU survivors had higher 3-year mortality (39.5%) than hospital controls (34.5%). ICU subjects who had received mechanical ventilation had substantially increased mortality at 3 years (57.6%). Most of the ventilated subjects died in the first 6 months after ICU admission (30.1% vs 9.6% for hospital controls). They concluded that an increase in mortality was present for 3 years after ICU admission.

In Australia, Williams and associates looked at all adult subjects admitted to the ICU who survived to hospital discharge.[2] They noted the risk of death for these subjects was higher than the general public for 15 years after ICU admission. They concluded that an episode of critical illness, or its treatment, may shorten life expectancy.

The author has nothing to disclose.
3835 Bosworth Drive, Roanoke VA, 24010, USA
E-mail address: ctoevs@aol.com

Surg Clin N Am 91 (2011) 325–331
doi:10.1016/j.suc.2010.12.008
0039-6109/11/$ – see front matter © 2011 Elsevier Inc. All rights reserved.

In Germany, Schneider and colleagues[3] looked specifically at long-term survival after surgical critical illness. They followed 1462 subjects with an ICU stay of greater than 4 days, until the end of the second year after ICU admission. Of the 1055 subjects (72.0%) discharged from the ICU, 808 (55.3%) survived 6 months, and at 2 years 648 (44.3%) subjects were alive. They concluded that survivors of surgical critical illness suffer from a post-ICU syndrome. They stated, "specific sequelae of critical illness may create a defined constellation of signs and symptoms that are both directly attributable to the episode of preceding critical illness and responsible for morbidity and mortality beyond the underlying disease."[3]

Dialysis is a frequent intervention started in the intensive care unit setting. As the population grows older, so does the age of patients in the ICU; more patients are being admitted from nursing home settings. Tamura and colleagues[4] studied hospitalized subjects in nursing homes with end-stage renal disease and the initiation of dialysis. At 12 months after initiation of dialysis, 58% of these subjects had died and predialysis functional status was maintained in only 13%. These were subjects with single-organ failure at the start of dialysis. Often ICU patients have multiple-organ failure, of which renal failure is just one component, supporting the poor outcome of initiation of dialysis in this patient population.

In Norway, Halverson[5] recommends that discussions about starting dialysis in the elderly population should involve the health care team and patients. He suggests a transparent discussion, involving the difficult decisions of withdrawing and withholding dialysis, should occur before initiation of dialysis. He also states that medicine tends to focus on the technical aspects of dialysis and neglects the overall needs of patients. Furthermore, consent involves only the technical components of the procedure and not in the context of overall outcomes of patients. This trend of technical procedural-based consent, rather than contextual informed context, is more common in elderly patients because the complexities of their needs are greater than younger patients.

Increasingly, hospitals and ICUs have been using long-term acute care hospitals (LTACs) to facilitate recovery from a critical illness. However, the outcomes of these patients being transferred to LTACs are rarely communicated to the patients and families. The 1-year survival of Medicare beneficiaries transferred to an LTAC is 52%.[6] In their study, Kahn and associates commented that we need strategies "to improve both prognosis and communication about prognosis to ensure decision makers do not have unreasonable expectations surrounding long-term acute care."[6]

Regarding trauma patients specifically, in New Jersey, Livingston and associates[7] evaluated the long-term outcomes of trauma subjects admitted to the SICU. They contacted 100 subjects who experienced trauma with ICU stays greater than 10 days. A total of 81 subjects were men with a mean age of 42 years. Traumatic brain injury was present in 50 subjects. The mean follow-up was 3.3 years from discharge. They noted that only 49% of subjects were back to work or school following injury. They noted ICU survivors greater than 3 years after severe injury have significant impairments, including inability to return to work. They stated, "The goal of reintegrating patients back into society is not being met." They concluded that although survival is an important outcome after injury, it is not a sufficient outcome to measure success of a trauma center.

DO NOT RESUSCITATE AND THE ICU

Physicians tend not to discuss do-not-resuscitate (DNR) orders with their patients. In New York, Sulmasy[8] surveyed doctors about their attitudes and confidence regarding DNR discussions. They noted physician confidence regarding DNR discussion is low compared with other medical discussions, such as procedural consent. They concluded that this lack of confidence in physicians having these discussions may contribute to the low occurrence rate of these conversations. Their study again supports the data that physicians' conversations with families tend to focus on technical aspects of treatment as opposed to long-term outcomes and contextual conversations based on goals of care.

Cardiopulmonary resuscitation (CPR) in an ICU setting is rarely effective in providing long-term survival and survival to hospital discharge. Myrianthefs and colleagues[9] looked at subjects (111 total) who underwent CPR in an adult ICU. The 24-hour survival of subjects was 9.2%. The survival to discharge was 0. They recommended that DNR orders should be applied more frequently in the ICU.

Surgical services tend to discuss DNR less frequently than medical services. Morrell and colleagues[10] in Indiana compared the use of DNR orders in medical subjects versus surgical subjects at time of hospital death. They noted DNR orders were more frequent on medical subjects (77.3%) than surgical subjects (64.2%). This study showed these orders were made earlier in the hospital stay for medical subjects (9.8 days before death) rather than for surgical subjects (5.1 days before death). They concluded that DNR orders are typically written late in the patients' hospital course on both medical and surgical services. They also noted several previous studies, in which DNR orders in subjects who died were written within 3 days of the subjects' deaths. They concluded that physicians still are reluctant to have these emotional and time-intensive conversations with patients and their families, thus contributing to the palliative medicine initiative.

END-OF-LIFE CARE IN SICU AND TRAUMA

In 2008, the American Academy of Critical Care Medicine published a consensus statement on their recommendations for end-of-life (EOL) care in the ICU.[11] They recommended intensivists should be competent in all aspects of end-of-life care, including the "practical and ethical aspects of withdrawing different modalities of life-sustaining treatment and the use of sedatives, analgesics and nonpharmacologic approaches to easing the suffering of the dying process." Evidence supports "improved communication with the family has been shown to improve patient care and family outcomes."[11]

Communication in the ICU around EOL issues remains problematic. Lautrette and colleagues[12] reviewed the literature regarding end-of-life family conferences. They noted multiple studies demonstrating proactive interventions are needed to improve communication at the end of life. They note families want better communication because improved communication improves the care of patients. They state these studies show families need more support than informal family conferences. Families require assistance in understanding the information provided, support during the decision-making process, and assistance with alleviating their guilt. Families also require assistance with achieving consensus among family members even when a health care proxy has been designated. These family meetings are time intensive, supporting the role of teams dedicated to patient and family support.

Part of the problem may lie in the ICU model of open versus closed intensive care units. Cassell and colleagues[13] looked at the comparison of administrative models of ICUs and the interactions of medical personnel and families. They noted that when surgeons have primary responsibility for patients, the most important goal is "defeating death."[13] When intensivists have sole patient responsibility (closed ICU model) then quality of life and scarcity of resources are considered. Their conclusions state the administrative models of ICU care need to be evaluated. Physician behavior will not change until the ICU model of care is addressed regardless of education of EOL principles.

One suggestion to improve communication in the ICU is a simple checklist on ICU admission. Mularski[14] proposed a checklist that would identify surrogate decision makers and explore goals of care from a patient-family perspective. Application and quality could be measured by increased documentation of patient goals and preferences in the medical record. A checklist, however, does not ensure that difficult and emotional conversations occur and that information is appropriately relayed to patients and families. Often, a more structured team approach as provided by palliative care services is needed in this process.

INTEGRATION OF A PALLIATIVE CARE TEAM

The medical intensive care unit (MICU) has already begun to investigate integrating the palliative medicine team into the ICU in certain situations. Campbell and Guzman,[15] at Wayne State University in Detroit, Michigan, compared ICU patients with end stage dementia who had a palliative medicine consult with those patients who did not have a palliative medicine consult. They noted a decreased hospital and MICU length of stay in subjects proactively identified with dementia and provided consultation from palliative medicine. They also noted that a "proactive palliative intervention decreased the time between identification of poor prognosis and the establishment of DNR goals, decreased time terminal demented subjects remained in the ICU, and reduced the use of nonbeneficial resources."[15] They stated that these interventions resulted in reduced burden and cost of care to the subjects and their families with increasing comfort and psycho-emotional support. There was no difference in the mortality or discharge to nursing home versus home in the 2 groups. In their study, palliative medicine consultation resulted in decreased length of stay and shorter time to defining goals of care without increasing mortality.

A similar study was done in the MICU in Rochester, New York. Norton and her team identified 191 subjects who, on admission to the MICU, had a high risk of dying.[16] Two-thirds of these subjects had palliative care consultation. Their data showed that subjects in the palliative care consultation group had a significantly shorter length of stay in the MICU, without a difference in total length of stay in the hospital. There were no differences in mortality rates or discharge disposition between the groups. They concluded that there is a growing body of literature suggesting that "proactive interventions focused on enhancing communication regarding patients' goals of care and benefits verses burdens of treatment are associated with shortened lengths of stay"[16] in the ICU.

In New York, O'Mahony and colleagues[17] published a descriptive study of the logistics of integration of the palliative care team into the ICUs at their hospitals. The advance practice nurse on the palliative care team went to the ICU daily to communicate with the ICU team. The palliative care team was consulted on one-third of the subjects that ultimately died within the ICU. They noted that subjects and families who had a consult had increased communication, education on the death process, improvements in pain and symptom management, increase in formalization of advance directives, and decrease in laboratory and radiology tests. Survival times were identical between the subjects that had palliative care involvement verses those who did not.

The SICU in Milwaukee tried to establish the use of triggers for increasing access to palliative care. Bradley and colleagues[18] identified subjects who would benefit from palliative care consultation as those who had a family request, futility considered or declared by medical team, family disagreement lasting more than 7 days, death expected during the same SICU stay, SICU stay greater than 1 month, diagnosis with median survival less than 6 months, greater than 3 SICU admissions during same hospitalization, Glasgow Coma Scale of less than 8 for more than 1 week in subjects aged younger than 75 years, and multiorgan failure in greater than 3 systems. Despite these triggers and identification of these subjects, the consult was at the discretion of the primary service or the SICU service in this ICU model. They noted that the use of triggers successfully identifies the subjects who were at a high risk of poor outcome (>50% mortality). However, the use of palliative care consults did not increase during the time period the triggers were implemented because the consult was optional and not mandatory. They suggested the daily use of a "palliative care bundle"[18] by the SICU team that addresses symptom control, goal setting and prognostication, psychosocial and spiritual support, advance care planning, and patient and family support, may improve outcomes for the patients in the SICU. They also suggested this bundle may work best in a closed ICU model.

Even with trauma patients in the ICU, a structured approach to palliative intervention was found to be beneficial. In New Jersey, Mosenthal and associates[19] instituted a palliative program implemented by the trauma surgeons and ICU nursing. This program included, on admission to the SICU, family bereavement support and assessment of prognosis and patient preferences. Secondly, they implemented interdisciplinary family meetings within 72 hours of admission. They noted the implementation of a palliative program did not change mortality, DNR, or withdraw of life-sustaining therapy rates, but both DNR and withdraw were implemented earlier in the hospital course. Of the patients who died, the ICU length of stay was decreased, and the time from DNR order to death was increased. They concluded that structured communication between physicians and families resulted in earlier consensus around goals of care for dying trauma patients. Integrating an early structured palliative program resulted in improved communication with families and improvement of EOL care.

The University of Rochester Medical Center launched an initiative to provide early consultation with palliative care for patients with severe traumatic brain injury.[20] They noted earlier and more thorough discussions with families about prognosis, patients' values, and outcomes occurred after routine palliative care consultation. They noted a small but significant decrease in tracheostomies performed in this patient population and an increase in withdraw of mechanical ventilation before tracheostomy. They noted that the integration of a palliative care team resulted in increased conversations with families "about the delicate, complex and emotionally demanding decisions required to achieve fully informed choice in life-changing, unfamiliar and often terrifying situations." They also noted medicine needs to move toward "more systematic conversations about the potential for invasive medical treatments both to do good and to harm patients toward the end of life."[20]

Recommendations for improving the quality of EOL care have been proposed by Nelson.[21] She stated the goals of integrating palliative care in the ICU are to optimize comfort and function for patients at all stages of serious and life-threatening disease. Integrating palliative care on admission to the ICU provided emotional and practical support for families, beginning at diagnosis of critical illness, regardless of prognosis. In this model, palliative care is part of comprehensive critical care, not as an optional alternative, and is simultaneous with critical care rather than sequential. Patients can continue treatments with the goal of restoring health, and there is not an expectation that critical illness will result in death. Rather than trying to change the attitudes in society and medicine toward death, the emphasis is on transforming the experience of dying in the ICU.

SUMMARY

As the population ages, the age of patients within the ICU also increases. In many of these clinical situations of trauma and postoperative surgical care, we do not adequately address the goals of care with patients and their families. An early integrated approach of palliative medicine in the SICU and trauma would offer patients and families improved communication of goals of care and support. Identification of evidence-based triggers for palliative medicine consults would facilitate this process (dialysis, tracheostomy in traumatic brain injury, dementia, ventilator >7 days, and so forth). Palliative medicine in the ICU offers the opportunity to decrease length of stay and decrease nonbeneficial resource use without increasing mortality. Taking care of our patients and their families and addressing all of their needs and goals, not just the physical, should be the role of every intensivist and trauma surgeon.

ACKNOWLEDGMENTS

The author sincerely thanks Ellen Harvey, MN, RN, CCRN, CNS, for her editorial assistance.

REFERENCES

1. Wunsch H, Guerra C, Barnato A, et al. Three-year outcomes for Medicare beneficiaries who survive intensive care. JAMA 2010;303:849–56.
2. Williams T, Dobb G, Finn J, et al. Determinants of long-term survival after intensive care. Crit Care Med 2008;36:1523–30.
3. Schneider C, Fertmann J, Geiger S, et al. Long-term survival after surgical critical illness: the impact of prolonged preceding organ support therapy. Ann Surg 2010;251:1145–53.
4. Tamara M, Covinsky K, Chertow G, et al. Functional status of elderly adults before and after initiation of dialysis. N Engl J Med 2009;361:1539–47.
5. Halvorsen k, Slettebo A, Nortbedt P, et al. Priority dilemmas in dialysis: the impact of old age. J Med Ethics 2008;34:585–9.
6. Kahn J, Benson N, Appleby D, et al. Long-term acute care hospital utilization after critical illness. JAMA 2010;303:2253–9.
7. Livingston D, Tripp T, Biggs C, et al. A fate worse than death? Long-term outcome of trauma patients admitted to the surgical intensive care unit. J Trauma 2009;67: 341–9.
8. Sulmasy D, Sood J, Ury W. Physicians' confidence in discussion do not resuscitate orders with patients and surrogates. J Med Ethics 2008;34:96–101.
9. Myrianthefs P, Kalafati M, Lemonidou C, et al. Efficacy of CPR in a general adult ICU. Resuscitation 2003;57:43–8.
10. Morrell E, Brown B, Qi R, et al. The do-not-resuscitate order: associations with advance directives, physician specialty and documentation of discussion 15 years after the Patient Self-Determination Act. J Med Ethics 2008;34:642–7.
11. Truog R, Campbell M, Curtis J, et al. Recommendation for end-of-life care in the intensive care unit: a consensus statement by the American Academy of Critical Care Medicine. Crit Care Med 2008;36:953–63.

12. Lautrette A, Ciroldi M, Ksibi H, et al. End-of-life family conferences: rooted in the evidence. Crit Care Med 2006;34(Suppl):S364–72.

13. Cassell J, Buckman T, Streat S, et al. Surgeons, intensivists, and the covenant of care: administrative models and values affecting care at the end of life. Crit Care Med 2003;31:1263–70.

14. Mularski R. Defining and measuring quality palliative and end-of-life care in the intensive care unit. Crit Care Med 2006;34(Suppl):S309–16.

15. Campbell M, Guzman J. A proactive approach to improve end-of-life care in a medical intensive care unit for patients with terminal dementia. Crit Care Med 2004;32:1839–43.

16. Norton S, Hogan L, Holloway R, et al. Proactive palliative care in the medical intensive care unit: effects on length of stay for selected high-risk patients. Crit Care Med 2007;35:1530–5.

17. O'Mahony S, McHenry J, Blank A, et al. Preliminary report of the integration of a palliative care team into an intensive care unit. Palliat Med 2010;24:154–65.

18. Bradley C, Weaver J, Brasel K. Addressing access to palliative care services in the surgical intensive care unit. Surgery 2010;147:871–7.

19. Mosenthal A, Murphy P, Barker L, et al. Changing the culture around end-of-life care in the trauma intensive care unit. J Trauma 2008;64:1587–93.

20. Holloway R, Quill T. Treatment decisions after brain injury – tensions among quality, preference and cost. N Engl J Med 2010;362:1757–9.

21. Nelson J. Identifying and overcoming the barriers to high-quality palliative care in the intensive care unit. Crit Care Med 2006;34(Suppl):S324–31.

Care of the Family in the Surgical Intensive Care Unit

Leslie Steele Tyrie, MD[a], Anne Charlotte Mosenthal, MD[b],*

KEYWORDS

- Surgical intensive care unit • Palliative care • Family support
- Surrogate decision maker • Communication

One of the subtle but important shifts in surgical palliative care from usual surgical care is the treatment of the family and patient as the unit of care. Nowhere is this more apparent than in the surgical intensive care unit (SICU), where the stress of having a critically ill loved one creates significant bereavement and emotional needs for family members. Multiple studies have now demonstrated that families of patients in the ICU are themselves in crisis, with high levels of stress, anxiety, and depression regardless of whether the patient lives or dies.[1–4] Family perception of the patient's distress and suffering can also contribute to this. Families are usually called on to be surrogate decision makers for the patient in the ICU, further adding to their burden and emotional needs. The availability of emotional support, information, and appropriate communication for family not only affects their level of distress while in the ICU, but can predict their long-term bereavement and psychosocial outcome and whether or not they develop posttraumatic stress disorder (PTSD), anxiety, or depression.[5,6] How this affects the surviving patient's long-term outcome in turn is not clear, but one can speculate that patient and family distress are interrelated. Standard surgical ICU care must include both interdisciplinary teams and processes of care that specifically address the needs of patients' families with respect to communication, emotional support, information, and decision making.[7,8] If the ICU stay results in the death of the patient, appropriate end-of-life care should also include further support for families in bereavement, decision making, cultural observances, and ample access and time to be at the patient's bedside.

THE FAMILY EXPERIENCE IN THE SICU: GRIEF AND BEREAVEMENT

Grief is a normal but profound emotional reaction to the loss of a loved one. Grief includes diverse emotional, behavioral, cognitive, and physiologic manifestations

[a] Department of Surgery, New Jersey Medical School, University of Medicine and Dentistry of New Jersey, 185 South Orange Avenue, MSB G506, Newark, NJ 07103, USA
[b] Trauma/Critical Care Division, University Hospital - New Jersey Medical School, 150 Bergen Street, Mezz 233, Newark, NJ 07103, USA
* Corresponding author.
E-mail address: mosentac@umdnj.edu

Surg Clin N Am 91 (2011) 333–342
doi:10.1016/j.suc.2011.01.003
0039-6109/11/$ – see front matter © 2011 Elsevier Inc. All rights reserved.

surgical.theclinics.com

(**Box 1**). Families may manifest grief in some or all of these ways, at different times, and with different intensity. How families cope with grief will affect their behavior and interactions with the ICU team and the patient. More importantly, how the SICU team supports and interacts with families will have a profound impact on both their acute and long-term bereavement. Grief occurs not only after death, but after any major loss. Even if the patient survives the SICU stay, but has permanent disability, grief may complicate both the patient's and family's recovery. Medical events such as anoxic brain injury, stroke, amputation, or spinal cord injury leading to permanent loss of function mean loss of hopes, expectations, and life as previously known. Such a situation can be devastating—families and patients will experience the same sequence of grief and coping mechanisms as is apparent after a death.

In a surgical or trauma ICU the family may be facing the death of a loved one suddenly and without warning, while in other cases the critical illness may follow a long period of chronic illness and disability with significant stress on families as

---

Box 1
Manifestations of grief

Emotional
- Despair
- Anxiety
- Guilt
- Anger
- Hostility
- Loneliness

Behavioral
- Agitation
- Fatigue
- Crying
- Social withdrawal

Cognitive
- Decreased self-esteem
- Preoccupation with the image of deceased
- Helplessness
- Hopelessness
- Self-blame
- Problems with concentration

Physiologic
- Anorexia
- Sleep disturbances
- Energy loss and exhaustion
- Somatic complaints
- Susceptibility to illness/disease

caregivers even before the ICU admission. If the ICU admission follows a transplant or oncologic surgery, families may have high hopes and expectation for life-changing surgery and "rescue." If these hopes are not met, families have difficulty coping with this reality, and may be further overwhelmed. Even if patients die after weeks or months of a long illness, to families this is still a sudden and acutely disruptive event. Their experience of the ICU stay, while "routine" for the staff, may be one of turbulence, uncertainty, and hope alternating with despair, all depending on the condition of the patient; families become exhausted, ignoring their own needs for rest and food. Families have probably coped with emotional distress and impending loss using the defense of denial. Death of the patient now shatters that defense. In all of these scenarios grief will be manifest as anger, denial, blame, anxiety, and sorrow.

The ability of families to cope with grief is affected by the social and cultural context in which they live, the nature and availability of support systems,[9] previous loss, and their coping styles. Sudden death or death related to trauma or violence may complicate the ability to cope. Increasing evidence suggests that death in the ICU is experienced as traumatic for many families, and their bereavement is complicated in a similar way, if they are not supported.[1,4,10,11] Grief and bereavement theory suggests several reasons for this that are relevant to care of families in the SICU (**Box 2**).

FAMILY AS SURROGATE DECISION MAKER

Twenty percent of patient deaths in the United States occur in the ICU.[12] Ninety percent of deaths in the ICU occur after decisions to withhold or withdraw life-sustaining treatments; however, fewer than 5% of ICU patients have sufficient capacity to make their own decisions about care.[13] Only 10% of ICU patients have advance directives, though advance directives may still not clearly elucidate the nuances of which plan of care would be desired by the patient.[14] These difficult decisions regarding treatment limitation and life support are left to be made by surrogates—the patients' families. Families already under stress due to grief and emotional distress may be further stressed when asked to be the surrogate decision makers; this can interfere with patient care and medical decision making, depending on the ability of families to cope. Complicated grief of the family can lead to conflict within families or with the medical team, prolonging end-of-life care and undermining decision making for the patient. Conversely, when stressed families are asked to understand sophisticated medical information and make life and death decisions for

---

Box 2
Experiences of grief by patient families in the SICU

- The shock of the death overwhelms the self and diminishes ability to cope.
- The perception of the world as orderly and meaningful is shattered, leading to intense reactions of fear, anxiety, and loss of control.
- The mourner experiences a profound loss of security and confidence in the world causing increased anxiety.
- The loss does not make sense and cannot be absorbed.
- There is no chance to say goodbye, leaving unfinished business with the deceased.
- Families have a strong need to determine blame and affix responsibility for it.
- The loss highlights events around the time of death, distorting recollections of the relationship with the deceased and causing survivor guilt.

another, the role of surrogate not only becomes an unwanted burden, but compounds their own grief and distress. Their ability to cope with grief and bereavement can become further impaired, just when the patient's care needs them most. One-third to one-half of families show signs of depression, anxiety, and posttraumatic stress symptoms while their loved one is in the ICU.[1,3,4,10] These emotional factors are more apparent if the patient dies, but are most heightened if the families have participated in end-of-life decision making as a surrogate, or have experienced discordance or conflict in their decision-making role.[3,4,15] Several studies followed families after ICU discharge. Forty-two percent of families of ICU patients experienced significant anxiety, 16% experienced depression, and 35% had PTSD at 6 months after a loved one's death.[1] Family mental health scores in health-related quality of life assessments were impaired at 90 days after patient discharge; this was associated with end-of-life treatment limitation decisions as well as perceived conflict around care.[16] Families may confuse their involvement as surrogate decision makers, and believe that they are solely responsible for making life and death decisions. The presence of an advance directive, or a previous conversation with the patient about their preferences for treatment, can alleviate some of this burden for families. Although it has been shown that as they are currently used, advance directives do not affect the cost of ICU care and do not change ICU end-of-life decision making,[17] they are effective tools to guide both families and physicians and diminish long-term feelings of guilt, complicated grief, and distress.

While the family's role as surrogate is affected by grief and emotional stress, it can also be affected by their social and cultural community, life circumstances, and coping styles. The expectation in Western medicine that patient autonomy is the prevailing ethical principle may add additional stress to family members from cultures where elders, religious leaders, or male relatives would normally make important decisions. Sociologic study has revealed factors that can support or detract from family ability to function as a surrogate (**Table 1**).[18]

How families cope as surrogate decision makers is also affected by their perception of the critical illness and prognosis of the patient's condition. Families may not rely solely on physician prognostications or medical information in forming their opinions on the loved one's condition or chances for recovery. While in some cases this may reflect a lack of trust in the medical system, it is equally likely that it reflects beliefs

Table 1
Family social factors that affect role as surrogate

Helps	Hinders
Previous experiences as decision makers	Competing responsibilities in family
Presence of coping skills	Surrogate's poor health
Religious support Decisions that align with surrogate beliefs	Financial burdens
Support in friend/family network Sense of keeping a patient promise	Family conflicts
Sense that decision helps the patient (ie, avoid suffering) Feeling involved in patient care	Personal attachment to patient
Knowing patient preferences	Not knowing patient preferences

Adapted from Vig EK, Starks HS, Taylor JS, et al. Surviving surrogate decision-making: what helps and hampers the experience of making medical decisions for others. J Gen Intern Med 2007;22:1274–9.

about the patient's character, strength of will ("he's a fighter"), belief in miracles, or religious faith.[19] When asked to discuss a patient's chance of survival, both the critically ill and their surrogates predict a higher chance of survival then their actual survival rate or APACHE II predicted mortality.[20] There was no difference in families' understanding of prognostication or incorporation into goal setting if told prognostic information in numerical terms (ie, "Your father has a 10% chance of survival) versus descriptive terms (ie, "Your father is seriously ill"). In addition, after being told in these specific terms about likelihood of death, a patient's surrogate still perceived the chance of survival as higher than the physician's estimate.[21] Families' perception of illness among the critically ill is more influenced by their own emotional and cognitive beliefs—faith, sense of personal control, belief in success/failure of medical therapy— than by prognostications of physicians.[22,23] These perceptions, in turn, clearly will affect a family's ability to set appropriate goals of care and treatment plans for the patient. Key elements of their conceptualization and beliefs are described in **Box 3**.

A recent study suggests that when soliciting reactions to the aforementioned domains from patients and surrogates about their critical illness state, there are differences in perception between groups. African Americans were more likely to be optimistic about the illness but also felt they had less understanding of the disease when compared with Caucasians. In addition, the presence of Christian faith or activity in church was an independent predictor of belief that medical treatment would improve the illness course. African Americans and those patients who identify a strong faith or participation in church are two groups who are more likely to pursue aggressive care and are reluctant to withdraw life support.[24,25] Though not definitively shown, it is possible this treatment preference is related to perceptions about disease. While this remains an area for further study, we must acknowledge that the surrogate's perception of the patient's situation is influenced not only by medical facts but also by family beliefs and background regarding medical information.

WHAT DO FAMILIES NEED?

Much of the emotional and spiritual suffering around the end of life in the SICU is experienced by the family. Studies on breaking bad news after sudden death have shown that the manner in which death or poor outcome is relayed to the family can have life-long ramifications for their bereavement.[26] A survey of surviving families of trauma patients notes that the top 3 things they value in the care of their loved ones were a caring attitude of the news giver, the clarity of the message, and the opportunity

---

Box 3
Family factors affecting perception of illness and prognosis

- Chronologic course of illness (acute vs chronic)
- Likely outcome of illness
- Emotional impact of illness
- Sense of personal control over illness state
- Ability of medical care to improve illness state
- Perception of personal understanding

Data from Ford D, Zapka J, Gebregziabher M, et al. Factors associated with illness perception among critically ill patients and surrogates. Chest 2010;138:59–67.

to ask questions.[27] Family needs are more complex when death and dying occurs in the setting of treatment limitation options and surrogate decisions. Several studies have identified factors that positively affect surrogate decision-maker experience, and minimize family stress and iatrogenic suffering **Box 4**.[18]

Studies show that there are specific interventions that can positively affect the care of dying patients' families. The positive impact of hospital-based bereavement services, pastoral care, or family support personnel is becoming increasingly apparent on the long-term psychosocial functioning of surviving families and on other outcomes, such as organ donation.[28,29] Many interventions revolve around establishing a communication plan, providing written materials about the patient's condition, addressing end-of-life care early, and providing bereavement and emotional support. ICUs that have standard processes of care such as a "communication bundle" (ie, family meetings within 72 hours, emotional support within 24 hours) have a positive impact on family outcomes.[7,8] Setting up an intensive communication plan aimed at families, which provides emotional, educational, and decisional support, will establish therapeutic goals based on patient preferences *earlier*, decrease conflict, and decrease family distress, without a significant change in patient mortality.[30–34] In addition, family leaflets providing information regarding disease and treatment have been shown to improve comprehension and satisfaction among families with the capability to understand the medical care.[5,6] Finally, initiating discussion of end-of-life care both as education and support before decisions need to be made has been shown to alleviate stress, anxiety, and depression regarding these issues. Talking about end-of-life issues early provides families with a structured forum to expose their individual needs and concerns, as well as express any guilt they may have regarding being involved in end-of-life decision making.[26,32]

Box 4
Factors affecting family distress as surrogate decision makers

Decrease Distress

- Unlimited access to loved ones
- Family meetings, sense of clinician availability
- Privacy
- Communication involving a show of compassion, respect, listening, and honesty
- Hope, dignity, choice, and finding meaning in patient experience
- Patient comfort and free of suffering
- Frank information about condition and prognosis from clinicians
- Recommendations from clinicians
- Support for surrogate choices from clinicians

Increase Distress

- Lack of clear data or contradictory information
- Infrequent discussions or discussion in a busy place (ie, waiting room)
- Conflicts between team members

Data from Vig EK, Starks HS, Taylor JS, et al. Surviving surrogate decision-making: what helps and hampers the experience of making medical decisions for others. J Gen Intern Med 2007;22:1274–9.

PALLIATIVE CARE INTERVENTIONS TO SUPPORT FAMILIES IN THE ICU

To support families in the ICU both for bereavement and as surrogate decision makers requires systematic processes of care as well as an interdisciplinary team. Family satisfaction and long-term bereavement outcomes are improved with communication and emotional support interventions.[5,6,27,28,32,33] There are several keys to understanding the approach to successful family communication in the ICU setting. First, it is important to recognize communication as a defined process and skill with specific approaches to improve family satisfaction.[33,35] Just as there are a series of key steps for any procedure or algorithm, preparation is required for successful family communication. Second, families' readiness to accept bad news and their response to grief is also a process and takes time. While the patient in the ICU may be critically ill and need

---

Box 5
SPIKES: A 6-step protocol for delivering bad news

Step 1: S: Setting up the interview

- Arrange for privacy and a quiet place
- Involve key family members
- Sit down and introduce yourself
- Make connection with the family
- Manage time constraints and interruptions

Step 2: P: assessing the family's Perception

- Find out what the family already knows

Step 3: I: obtaining the family's Invitation

- Find out what the family wants to know

Step 4: K: giving Knowledge and information to the family

- Avoid medical jargon
- Give information in small amounts at a time
- Educate about patient's condition and prognosis
- Express uncertainty honestly

Step 5: E: addressing the family's Emotions with Empathetic responses

- Listen and respond to family's feelings
- Allow time for expression of emotion
- Identify family's emotion
- Identify cause of emotion
- Connect emotion with the cause of emotion

Step 6: S: Strategy and Summary

- Discuss goals of care
- Treatment plans
- Future meetings

Adapted from Buckman R. Communication in palliative care: a practical guide. In: Doyle D, Hanks GWC, McDonald N, editors. Oxford textbook of palliative medicine. 2nd edition. New York: Oxford University Press; 1998; p. 141–56.

immediate decisions to be made about the next step in care, families must be ready and willing to undertake the task of becoming decision makers, and this cannot be rushed despite the acuity of the patient's situation. It takes time to build a trusting and collaborative relationship with a patient's family. Several communication approaches that improve family satisfaction and outcomes have been well described.[32,35,36] The SPIKES protocol and the VALUE protocol are two examples. Buckman[36] outlined 6 steps to communicate bad news to patients' loved ones, and an adaptation for families is shown in **Box 5**.

Interdisciplinary communication both educates and supports the family. The whole ICU team should be involved in this process to prevent iatrogenic suffering of the family as much as possible. Several models of interdisciplinary communication have been shown to be effective as emotional and decisional support for families, especially in their role as surrogate decision maker.[4–6,30,31,34,37] The team should include the physician, the nurse, a psychosocial or bereavement support professional, and spiritual/pastoral care. While physicians provide expertise in medical information and prognosis, others can support the family particularly in their role as surrogate. Each member of the team has a different role, but many may have direct contact with patients and their families. Every member is a potential resource to a patient's family. Consensus among all caregivers is important not only for cohesive patient care but also for family care; families identify conflict within the medical team as one of the distressing aspects of care in the ICU.[18] Critical care nurses have wide exposure to a patient's loved ones. Families appear to receive important communication through nurses and rate their skill in communication as one of the more important in their experience.[38] Although nurses often have more access to patients' families and by the nature of that exposure are a key element of communication regarding patient care, there are data to suggest they are not inherently better at this communication than doctors.[39] This problem can be addressed by bringing all members of the team up to speed on patient prognosis and care goals during morning rounds or in a structured format. Nurses may benefit from training to specifically improve their communication skills.

REFERENCES

1. Anderson WG, Arnold RM, Angus DC, et al. Posttraumatic stress and complicated grief in family members of patients in the intensive care unit. J Gen Intern Med 2008;23(11):1871–6.
2. McAdam JL, Dracup KA, White DB, et al. Symptom experiences of families of intensive care unit patients. Crit Care Med 2010;38:1075–85.
3. Pochard F, Darmon M, Fassier T, et al. Symptoms of anxiety and depression in family members of intensive care unit patients before discharge or death. a prospective multicenter study. J Crit Care 2005;20:90–6.
4. Azoulay E, Pochard F, Kentish-Barnes N, et al. Risk of post-traumatic stress symptoms in family members of intensive care unit patients. Am J Respir Crit Care Med 2005;171:987–94.
5. Azoulay E, Pochard F, Chevret S, et al. Impact of a family information leaflet on effectiveness of information provided to family members of intensive care unit patients: a multicentre, prospective, randomized, controlled trail. Am J Respir Crit Care Med 2002;165:438–42.
6. Lautrette A, Darmon M, Megarbane B, et al. A communication strategy and brochure for relatives of patients dying in the ICU. N Engl J Med 2007;356:469–78.

7. Nelson JE, Brasel KJ, Campbell ML, et al. for the IPAL_ICU Project. Evaluation of ICU palliative care quality: a technical assistance monograph from the IPAL-ICU Project. Center to Advance Palliative Care 2010. [Epub ahead of print].

8. Robert D, Truog MA, Margaret L, et al. Recommendations for end-of-life care in the intensive care unit: a consensus statement by the American Academy of Critical Care Medicine. Crit Care Med 2008;36(3):953–63.

9. Rando T. Treatment of complicated mourning. Champaign (IL): Research Press; 1993.

10. Siegel M, Hayes E, Vandereweker L, et al. Psychiatric illness in the next of kin of patients who die in the ICU. Crit Care Med 2008;36:1722–5.

11. Van der Klink MA, Heijboer L, Hofhuis JG, et al. Survey into bereavement of family members of patients who died in the intensive care unit. Intensive Crit Care Nurs 2010;26:215–25.

12. Linde-Zwirble W, Angus DC, Griffin M, et al. ICU care at the end-of-life in America: an epidemiological study. Crit Care Med 2000;28:A34.

13. Prendergast TJ, Luce JM. Increasing incidence of withholding and withdrawal of life support from the critically ill. Am J Respir Crit Care Med 1997;155:15–20.

14. Danis M, Mutran E, Garrett JM, et al. A prospective study of the impact of patient preferences on life-sustaining treatment and hospital cost. Crit Care Med 1996; 24:1811–7.

15. Gries CJ, Engelberg RA, Kross EK, et al. Predictors of symptoms of posttraumatic stress and depression in family members after patient death in the ICU. Chest 2010;137:280–7.

16. Lemiale V, Kentish-Barnes N, Chaize M, et al. Health-related quality of life in family members of intensive care unit patients. J Palliat Med 2010;13:1131–7.

17. Teno JM, Lynn J, Wenger N, et al. Advance directives for seriously ill hospitalized patients: effectiveness with the patient self-determination act and the SUPPORT intervention. SUPPORT Investigators. Study to understand prognoses and preferences for outcomes and risks of treatment. J Am Geriatr Soc 1997; 45:500–70.

18. Vig EK, Starks HS, Taylor JS, et al. Surviving surrogate decision-making: what helps and hampers the experience of making medical decisions for others. J Gen Intern Med 2007;22:1274–9.

19. Boyd EA, Lo B, Evans LR, et al. "Its not just what the doctor tells me" factors that influences surrogate decision-makers' perceptions of prognosis. Crit Care Med 2010;38:1270–5.

20. Ford D, Zapka JG, Gebregziabher M, et al. Investigating critically ill patients' and families' perceptions of likelihood of survival. J Palliat Med 2009;12(1):45–52.

21. Lee Char SJ, Evans LR, Malvar GL, et al. A randomized trial of two methods to disclose prognosis to surrogate decision makers in intensive care units. Am J Respir Crit Care Med 2010;182(7):905–9.

22. Ford D, Zapka J, Gebregziabher M, et al. Factors associated with illness perception among critically ill patients and surrogates. Chest 2010;138:59–67.

23. Leventhal H, Meyer D, Nerenz DR. The common-sense representation of illness danger. In: Rachman S, editor. Medical psychology. New York: Pergamon; 1980. p. 7–30.

24. Hopp FP, Duffy SA. Racial variations in end-of-life-care. J Am Geriatr Soc 2000; 48:658–63.

25. Phelps AC, Maciejewski PK, Nilsson M, et al. Religious coping and use of intensive life-prolonging care near death in patients with advanced cancer. JAMA 2009;301:1140–7.

26. Iverson K. Grave words: notifying survivors about sudden unexpected deaths. Tucson (AZ): Galen Press; 1999.
27. Jurkevich GJ, Pierce B, Pananen L, et al. Giving bad news: the family perspective. J Trauma 2000;48:865–73.
28. Oliver RD, Sturtevant JP, Scheetz JP, et al. Beneficial effects of a hospital bereavement intervention program after traumatic childhood death. J Trauma 2001;50:440–8.
29. Linyear AS, Tartaglia A. Family communication coordination: a program to increase organ donation. J Transpl Coord 1999;9:165–74.
30. Lilly CM, De Meo DL, Sonna LA, et al. An intensive communication intervention for the critically ill. Am J Med 2000;109:469–75.
31. Mosenthal AC, Murphy PA, Barker LK, et al. Changing the culture of end of life care in the trauma ICU. J Trauma 2008;64(6):1587–93.
32. Curtis JR, Patrick DL, Shannon SE, et al. The family conference as a focus to improve communication about end-of-life care in the intensive care unit: opportunities for improvement. Crit Care Med 2001;29(Suppl 2):N26–33.
33. Curtis JR, Engelberg RA, Wenrich MD, et al. Missed opportunities during family conferences about end-of-life care in the intensive care unit. Am J Respir Crit Care Med 2005;171:844–9.
34. Schneiderman LJ, Gilmer T, Teetzel HD, et al. Effect of ethics consultations on nonbeneficial life-sustaining treatments in the intensive care setting: a randomized controlled trial. JAMA 2003;290:1166–72.
35. Stapleton RD, Engelberg RA, Wenrich MD, et al. Clinician statements and family satisfaction with family conferences in the intensive care unit. Crit Care Med 2006; 34:1679–85.
36. Buckman R. Communication in palliative care: a practical guide. In: Dereck D, editor. Oxford textbook of palliative medicine. 2nd edition. Oxford (England): Oxford University Press; 1998. p. 141–58.
37. Mcdonagh JR, Elliott TB, Engelberg RA, et al. Family satisfaction with family conferences about end of life care in the intensive care unit: increased proportion of family speech is associated with increased satisfaction. Crit Care Med 2004; 32:1484–8.
38. Hickey M. What are the needs of families of critically ill patients? A review of the literature since 1976. Heart Lung 1990;19:401–15.
39. Maguire PA, Faulkner A. Helping cancer patients disclose their concerns. Eur J Cancer 1996;32:78–81.

Palliative Surgical Oncology

Nader N. Hanna, MD[a],*, Emily Bellavance, MD[b],
Timothy Keay, MD[c]

KEYWORDS

- Palliative care • Surgical oncology • Ethics • Prognosis
- Cancer

A total of 1,529,560 new cancer cases and 569,490 deaths from cancer are projected to occur in the United States in 2010. The lifetime probability of being diagnosed with an invasive cancer is 44% for men and 38% for women. Advances in cancer treatment have lead to improvement in overall cancer survival rates, with the current 5-year relative survival rate of 68% for all cancers diagnosed in 1999 to 2005 (compared with 54% for all cancers diagnosed in 1984 to 1986). Approximately 10.8 million Americans with a history of cancer were alive in January 2004. The majority of cancer death is caused by progression of metastatic disease, and most cancer patients receive palliative treatment during their last few months of life.

Palliative surgical oncology is a relatively new concept, but builds on a long tradition in surgery. As the field of palliative medicine grows and becomes its own specialty, surgeons have been receiving some specialized training in palliative care; devising specific palliative surgical procedures; and reevaluating the ethics of their interactions with patients, especially for the selection of palliative surgical procedures. This is leading to a new form of surgical practice in which the emphasis is on relief of present or anticipated symptoms, even if the interventions do not prolong a patient's life span.

The objectives of this article are to (1) describe some of the history of palliative care related to the practice of surgical oncology, including educational efforts; (2) discuss goals and justifications for palliative surgery performed with the intent to alleviate existing symptoms and improve quality of life until death with less emphasis on overall patient survival; and (3) provide a discussion of ethical issues in palliative surgical oncology, especially as these relate to advance care planning and the maintenance of hope in the setting of cancer.

[a] Division of Surgical Oncology, University of Maryland School of Medicine, 22 South Greene Street, Suite S4B-12, Baltimore, MD 21201, USA
[b] Department of Surgery, University of Chicago, 5841 South Maryland Avenue, MC 5031, Chicago, IL 60637, USA
[c] Department of Family and Community Medicine, University of Maryland School of Medicine, 22 South Greene Street, Baltimore, MD 21201, USA
* Corresponding author.
E-mail address: nhanna@smail.umaryland.edu

Surg Clin N Am 91 (2011) 343–353
doi:10.1016/j.suc.2010.12.004
0039-6109/11/$ – see front matter © 2011 Elsevier Inc. All rights reserved.

WHAT IS PALLIATIVE CARE?

The very term "palliative care" was first put into use by a surgeon, Balfour Mount, MD, to describe a type of comprehensive, interdisciplinary, patient-centered care that provided symptom relief to dying patients.[1] Palliative care is the type of care currently delivered in the hospice insurance model of care as well as by independent palliative care services but has also been practiced by physicians and surgeons in most of their interventions for millennia.[2] The Billroth procedures, the Halsted radical mastectomies, the Whipple procedure, all were initially designed to provide a more peaceful and less symptomatic death in patients with terminal cancer. This palliative care tradition continues in the surgical exploration of new ways to enhance the care of patients with incurable illnesses, especially by focusing on the relief of present or imminent symptoms.

The basic domains of palliative care competency have been delineated in recent publications, especially in the development of a National Quality Forum's consensus statement on preferred practices for palliative care and hospice quality.[3] This forum divides the field into 8 domains, with 38 preferred practices, which provides a comprehensive overview of the field. The domains include areas such as structures of care, processes of care, physical aspects of care, psychological and psychiatric aspects of care, and care of the imminently dying patient. Surgical textbooks have to date provided only limited information on the topic of palliative care, although it is acknowledged that increasing the amount of information in these resources would be appropriate.[4] Recommendations for surgical competencies in specific areas, such as interpersonal and communication skills, have also been published.[5,6]

INTEGRATION OF RESIDENT/FELLOWS EDUCATION IN PALLIATIVE CARE INTO SURGICAL CURRICULUM

Education of surgeons in training about palliative care is an emerging field. There is consensus that a competent surgeon will have a basic level of skill in meeting the needs of all of those patients with life-threatening illnesses, including the dying patient. However, there is as yet no clear agreement as to the exact curricular needs or methods of teaching or evaluation. Different programs are experimenting with various teaching methods and curriculum so that their graduates will have improved their knowledge, attitudes, and skills in palliative care and provision of palliative surgical interventions. As noted by Galante and colleagues,[7] palliative care training is deficient in most postgraduate surgical training, yet could allow for the uniform and standard provision of palliative surgical care.

From the domains of palliative care, curricula have been developed for surgical education, and some of these curricula have been implemented. Brasel and Weissman[8] reviewed some of the educational programs for surgeons in 2004. Although they found many educational opportunities with overlapping topics of interest to surgeons, they found few actual educational programs specifically designed for surgery students or residents. They did note the barriers and the opportunities that existed, as well as some pilot programs that were being tried. In 2007, Weissman and colleagues[9] published the outcomes from a national multispecialty palliative care curriculum development project. Three hundred fifty eight residency programs in 4 specialties, including general surgery, participated in a palliative care curriculum development project, which resulted successfully in new teaching in pain management, nonpain symptom management, and communication skills. Focusing on the specific needs of surgeons, Brown University Medical School developed a surgical residency palliative care curriculum and published in 2007.[10] Their curriculum primarily focused on communication skills and decision making.

At the University of Maryland School of Medicine, the authors developed an online basic educational curriculum that was required for all Internal Medicine and Family Medicine first-year residents and all first-year Oncology fellows.[11,12] The authors are now implementing the new requirement of competency assessment tools for Internal Medicine residents to document palliative care skills.[13] To date, all of these online resources are used informally in surgical training at the University of Maryland, with mandatory completion being considered. The competencies are divided into 4 areas: (1) communication; (2) pain and symptom management; (3) ethical and legal aspects of care; and (4) psychosocial/cultural/spiritual aspects of care, hospice care, and referrals. Within these 4 areas, 19 competency assessment tools are available for directly observing and evaluating resident performance.

TEACHING PALLIATIVE CARE IN SURGICAL ONCOLOGY

The essence of all of these palliative care efforts seems to be "preservation of dignity," a topic explored by Chochinov.[14] Patients want to feel that they have hope, that they mean something to others, and that they receive the respect that is best summarized in the term "dignity." The word "dignity" should not be hijacked by those who want to promote physician-assisted suicide (eg, "Death with Dignity" organizations). Rather, a focus on dignity highlights the way in which the individual tools and skills to make a patient more comfortable are put together to provide a wholistic approach to a person with a life-threatening illness. The whole is truly greater than the sum of the parts when palliative care built around the concept of dignity is being provided to an individual person.

Role modeling by surgeons of the palliative approach to the patient as a person lies at the heart of all of palliative care education. This role modeling requires an attitude of caring for the person, behaviors that demonstrate respect, compassion that feels the suffering of the person without boundary disruption, and dialog for the provision of appropriate responses.[15] Thus, palliative care is not so much a new specialty, as a rediscovery of a tradition of surgery in which palliative surgical interventions that do not cure are once again acknowledged to be of tremendous benefit for those with disease.[16]

EVALUATION OF EDUCATION IN PALLIATIVE SURGICAL ONCOLOGY

Because the educational curriculum in palliative surgical oncology is so new, educational evaluation methods are not well established or standardized. The goal is to make palliative care "usual care" in advanced illness.[17] Therefore, outcome assessments are probably the most effective evaluation tools.

Chipman and colleagues[18] published their results describing the development and pilot testing of an Objective Structured Clinical Examination (OSCE) for leading family conferences in a surgical intensive care unit. They concluded that more work remained before this OSCE could be reliably used in summative evaluation. Also, this OSCE is not specifically designed for palliative oncology discussions but addressed such issues as general end-of-life discussion and disclosure of an iatrogenic complication. Another example of an outcome tool more specific to palliative oncology was provided by Helyer and colleagues[19] in their evaluation of surgeon's knowledge regarding gastric cancer surgery. Using a voluntary, mailed questionnaire, they found that most surgeons operating on gastric cancer in Ontario did not identify recommended quality indicators of gastric cancer surgery. They made several recommendations regarding continuing education to address this issue. Specific competency assessment tools for palliative surgical oncology are still lacking, however.

OBJECTIVES AND JUSTIFICATION FOR PALLIATIVE SURGICAL ONCOLOGY

The term "palliation" is derived from the Latin word *pallium*, which means to relieve or minimize. The definition of surgical palliation has evolved from the simple definition of noncurative surgery (due to residual or metastatic disease at completion of the operation or prophylactic to prevent development of anticipated symptoms) to surgery performed not to cure but to alleviate symptoms or restore organ function and offer the optimal quality of life until death. In the past, patients with advanced cancer were not provided with options for surgical palliation for many reasons. Patients were often considered to have untreatable terminal condition. Predominant therapeutic nihilism that has been the norm for these patients and surgery was often justified only by its potentially curative outcome. Palliative surgery was often cited to be associated with prolonged hospitalization, greater expense, and excessive morbidity and mortality. Surgery-induced stress and associated transient immune suppression were believed to result in physical dissemination and worsen prognosis. Most importantly, well-designed studies with precise definition of palliation, clear indications for palliative surgery, and proper outcome measures to evaluate the effectiveness of palliative surgery are lacking.

The primary objectives of surgical palliation include attainable and durable relief of symptoms and/or restoration of organ function and improve quality of life. Secondary objectives of palliative surgery may include improved response/effectiveness of additional therapies such as chemo/radiation and prolongation of quality-adjusted and progression-free survival. These benefits should be balanced against overall disease burden, other sites of metastatic disease, patient performance status, duration of hospitalization, surgical morbidity and mortality, anticipated survival, and need for additional palliative measures. Surgical oncologist for the most part have depended on their expertise in performing the most complex and challenging cancer surgeries and highest level of surgical judgment to carefully select patients that would benefit the most from palliative procedures rather than evidence-based data. Recent advances in surgical techniques, combination of surgical and nonsurgical palliative approaches, and the development of effective biologic and molecular-targeted therapies have led to paradigm shift in the role of palliative surgical oncology (**Table 1**).

Table 1	
Paradigm shift in role of palliative surgical oncology	
Conventional Practice	**New Concepts in Palliative Surgery**
Why?	Why not?
Terminal condition	Chronic disease
What are the resectability criteria	Unresectability criteria
Surgical limitation based on disease burden	Focus on preserving function of remnant organ
Morbidity/Mortality and long-term survival outcomes	Quality-adjusted survival and progression-free survival
Curative/Palliative	Cytoreduction/Debulking

In the authors' opinion, the best clinical outcomes and greatest patient satisfaction from palliative surgical oncology procedures can be achieved if the following conditions are considered:

A comprehensive palliative care plan is developed through multidisciplinary discussion of the patient condition and thorough understanding of the natural history of the disease.

Surgical palliation is judged to be the most effective intervention intended to provide durable alleviation of specific symptoms to justify the associated surgical morbidity.

The goals of the surgery to meet patient expectations are discussed.

Proper patient selection with at least 3-month expected survival and a Karnofsky performance status greater than 50%. Palliative surgery unlikely to be beneficial in patients who had exhausted all other treatment modalities.

Evaluating the outcomes of palliative surgical oncology is far from evidence-based with paucity of scientific data and controlled trials.[20] Palliative studies often consider different endpoints as a measure of success of surgical palliation. A study by Miner and colleagues[21] found that cost (2%), pain control (12%), quality of life (17%), need for repeated interventions (59%), surgical morbidity and mortality (61%), and survival (64%) are frequently reported as end-point success measures. A survey of members of the Society of Surgical Oncology showed that surgeons estimated 21% of their cancer surgeries as palliative in nature. Forty-three percent of respondents felt palliative surgery was best defined based on preoperative intent, 27% based on postoperative factors, and 30% based on patient prognosis. Only 43% considered estimated patient survival time an important factor in defining palliative surgery, yet 22% considered 5-year survival rate important.[22] Patient symptom relief and pain relief were identified as the 2 most important goals in palliative surgery, with increased survival being the least important.

The preservation of health-related quality of life (HRQoL) is an important goal of palliative treatment. Therefore, HRQoL should be an outcome measure in clinical trials of palliative treatment modalities.[23] Patient reported that quality of life measures eliminates the influence of physician bias, personal experience, and social or cultural environment. The timing of initial and interval assessment of outcomes after palliative surgery is crucial to the validation of quality of life outcomes and should take into account surgery-related factors (length of hospitalization, recovery duration, and treatment-related complications) and patient convenience and compliance. Therefore, a 6-week and 3-month postoperative assessment of quality of life and symptom response to the palliative procedure seems to offer a balanced response.

ETHICAL ISSUES IN PALLIATIVE SURGICAL ONCOLOGY

The contemporary practice of palliative care in surgical oncology includes a consideration of the ethical issues surrounding end-of-life decisions. While advances in technology have lead to prolonged life spans in critically and terminally ill patients, prolonging life at all costs is not always in the best interest of the patient. The physician-patient relationship has also changed in the past several decades from a relationship based on paternalism, to one focused on patient autonomy and shared decision making, further complicating ethical issues in palliative care. In a 2000 survey of Society of Surgical Oncology members, McCahill and colleagues[24] reported that the most common ethical dilemma encountered in palliative surgery was "providing patients with honest information without destroying hope," followed by preserving patient choice, use of advance directives, and withholding and withdrawing life-sustaining treatments. Thus, the surgical oncologist transitioning a patient from a curative to palliative care treatment plan can benefit from the consideration of common ethical issues encountered in palliative care.

DISCLOSING BAD NEWS

The honest disclosure of a poor or terminal prognosis is a well-established practice in the United States and is based on the ethical principles of autonomy and informed consent[25,26] and supported by legal precedent.[27] In practice, the principle of autonomy describes the right of patients to accept or decline medical treatment. An autonomous decision requires both intentionality and understanding on the part of patient and thus requires knowledge of relevant medical information. Truthful disclosure is also supported by the ethical principles of beneficence and nonmaleficence. Concealing a poor prognosis from a patient can erode trust developed in the doctor-patient relationship as well as prevent the patient and family members from preparing financially and emotionally for a poor outcome or death. However, transitioning a patient from a curative to palliative treatment plan remains a difficult task for both patient and physician. The responsibility to initiate this transition often falls on the shoulders of the surgical oncologist in the setting of unresectable cancer, disease progression that precludes further surgical or medical therapy, or life-threatening perioperative complications.

One helpful evidence-based template designed to guide clinicians in the disclosure of bad news is the "SPIKES" protocol.[28] The protocol consists of 6 basic steps following the "SPIKES" acronym: **S**etting up the interview, assessing the patient's **P**erception, obtaining the patient's **I**nvitation, giving **K**nowledge and information to the patient, addressing the patient's **E**motions with empathetic responses, and providing a **S**trategy and **S**ummary for the next steps for treatment. Setting up the interview can include such simple measures as arranging for privacy, asking the patient whether he or she would like significant others present for the discussion, and minimizing interruptions. Assessing the patient's perception of his or her medical condition allows the physician to clarify misunderstanding, assess for denial, and tailor the information to be given. Similarly, asking the patient to express how much or how detailed the patient desires the information to be at the first interview can allow the patient receive information in such a way that enables the patient to understand and process complex and disheartening information. Establishing the nature and amount of medical information that the patient desires early on in the conversation also allows the physician to identify the rare circumstance in which, for cultural or other personal reasons, the patient desires not to exercise his or her autonomy and effectively transfers the responsibilities of receiving information and making medical decision to a family member or other appointee. In both giving knowledge and summarizing a strategy, the physician can introduce a palliative care plan. Although the goals of the treatment have changed from cure or the temporal extension of life to goals of symptom control and the enhancement of quality of life, reassuring the patient that he or she will still be cared for can alleviate fears of abandonment. It is also in the establishment of these new palliative goals, as well as in the details of a palliative treatment plan, that the hope lies.

Based on qualitative data collected from interviews and observations of elderly cancer patients and terminally ill persons, Dufault and Martocchio[29] described hope as a dynamic process, defined by a "confident yet uncertain expectation of achieving a future good ... which is realistically possible and personally significant." According to this model, hope can be generalized as a sense of some beneficial, but unspecific future developments, or particularized and associated with an abstract or concrete specific goal. In cancer care, generalized hope may apply to the hope for quality of life or strength to endure, whereas particularized hope points to a specific outcome, such as the hope for cure or prolongation of life.[30] However, as the disease process evolves and the prognosis changes, the hopes can evolve and change. One of the most critical questions to be asked in a discussion introducing palliative care is, "If time becomes short, what is most important to you?"[31] The patient's answer to this question can guide the clinician in helping the patient achieve his or her goals, whether the goal is to spend quality time with family or, perhaps more concretely, to undergo successful treatment for intractable vomiting from a malignant bowel obstruction. Therefore, the process of honestly disclosing a poor prognosis and transitioning from curative to palliative care plan is not necessarily a hopeless endeavor.

ADVANCE DIRECTIVES

Advance directives are documents or verbal instructions used for the purpose of ensuring that a patient's wishes regarding end-of-life care are honored. Most of the patients will lose decision-making capacity at the end of life,[32] rendering advance directives a critical resource in preserving patient autonomy. Advance directives can be formal, as in a living will document or a durable power of attorney (DPA), or informal, manifest as verbal communication to family or friends. Although advance directives can be helpful guides when the patient is unable to articulate his or her desires about medical care, they are often fraught with difficulties because of ambiguity or disagreement among family members. Oftentimes, living wills make vague references to "no reasonable expectation of recovery," as the threshold for withdrawing life-sustaining treatments, rather than directing the clinician toward which specific treatments and outcomes are acceptable or unacceptable to the patient. Even if specific treatments such as hemodialysis or parenteral nutrition are referenced, these restrictions or allowances may be outdated as preferences can change with time or as the patient's medical condition evolves. Ideally, advance directives should be revisited with the patient over time with family members or a physician with whom the patient has a long-term relationship. The patient's primary care physician or medical oncologist may also be a helpful resource in the acute setting when there are questions regarding a patient's wishes expressed in an advance directive.

Expressing advance directives via a DPA can avoid some of the limitations of a written living will. However, controversies between family members can still arise, which may delay or inhibit care. Legally, medical decisions made by the DPA should be adhered to. Nonetheless, it is the physician's ethical duty to ensure that the medical decisions being made are in accordance with what the patient would have wanted. If the physician believes that the DPA's decisions are not in the best interest of the patient or do not reflect the patient's wishes, an attempt should be made to resolve this inconsistency. In these cases, it may be helpful to involve an ethics committee consultation, reserving legal action as a last resort.

WITHHOLDING AND WITHDRAWING LIFE-SUSTAINING TREATMENT

Many physicians find withdrawing life-sustaining treatment more difficult than withholding treatment.[33] The distinguishing factor between withdrawing and withholding treatment is the need for human agency in withdrawal.[34] A physician or member of the health care team is required to disconnect a ventilator or turn off vasopressor support. In addition, physicians seem to exhibit preferences in which interventions are acceptable to withdraw, preferring to withdraw treatments that support acute, rather than chronic, organ failure or treatments for an underlying disease process, rather than for an iatrogenic complication.[33] However, from a bioethical perspective, there is little distinction between withholding and withdrawing life-sustaining treatments.[35] Once a treatment is validly refused, by a patient or appropriate proxy, the treatment must not be started or must be withdrawn. Similarly, if a medical or surgical treatment is inappropriate, either because the treatment has no valid medical benefit or is inconsistent with the patient's goals of care, it should not be offered or should be stopped.

Most patients, at the end of their life are unable to contribute to the decision to withdraw or withhold life-sustaining treatments.[32] Although advance directives can be helpful guides for clinicians and family members, less than 30% of the adult population in the United States has prepared formal advance directives.[36] When a patient is unable to make medical decisions due to medical or cognitive incapacity, a surrogate decision maker must be appointed to act on the patient's behalf. Most states have legislature in place for prioritizing, according to familial relationship, the designation of a surrogate decision maker in the absence of an advance directive. In order to preserve patient autonomy, the surrogate should act according to the principle of substituted judgment, that is, to make decisions based on what the surrogate's best estimation of what the patient's wishes would be. Emphasizing that the surrogate's role is to articulate the patient's previously stated or inferred wishes, rather than to make independent decisions about a loved one's medical care, can help to alleviate some of the family's feelings of over-whelming responsibility and guilt when the decision is to proceed with comfort care in favor of life-sustaining measures. Similarly, in situations where family members disagree about end-of-life decisions, focusing the conversation on what *the patient would have wanted* can, over time, resolve controversies. When the patient's wishes are truly unknown, the surrogate's decisions should rely on the ethical principles of beneficence and nonmaleficence, that is, based on the best interests of the patient.

FUTILITY

A common problem encountered in the discussion of withdrawing life-sustaining treatment occurs when the surrogates, family members, or patients insist on continuing a treatment that the physician believes to be futile. Using medical futility as an ethical and legal argument to justify the unilateral withdrawal of life-sustaining treatments against a family or surrogate's wishes is laden with difficulties. The concept of medical futility carries both quantitative and qualitative connotations. There is little, if any, agreement among health care professionals on what numeric threshold of probable failure defines a futile intervention. More general definitions of futility describing a therapy as simply unlikely to meet with success allow for considerable variations among clinicians, who may determine that a treatment is futile if it carries a less than a 50% chance of success.

The term medical futility also carries a qualitative meaning implying that the objective of the treatment is not worthwhile.[37] Patients and their families may disagree with physicians on what defines a worthwhile outcome. Declaring a treatment to be futile may also further marginalize patients and surrogates by effectively negating their participation in future decision making. The ambiguities surrounding the concept of medical futility have lead some bioethicists to propose that the term "futility" be replaced by the terms "medically inappropriate" or "surgically inappropriate" to more accurately describe an assessment that reflects a professional opinion rather than a summation of value.[38]

Ultimately, a compromise must be reached between health care providers and the patient (or proxy) in determining what interventions are worthwhile. When there is disagreement about what the physician believes is overly aggressive care, it is essential to again revisit the question, "what is most important to the patient?" It is in defining an acceptable balance between the burdens and benefits of a proposed treatment with the patient or family members that a compromise can be reached. Occasionally, for personal or religious reasons, family members or patients may define the extension of life as the only acceptable end point even when death is imminent. Although there is some controversy about what to do in these cases, most physicians would find it difficult not to honor these rare requests to respect the patient's autonomy.

SUMMARY

The decision to perform a palliative surgical oncology procedure in a symptomatic patient is a frequent challenge for surgical oncologists and requires a high level of surgical judgment and surgical expertise. Surgical palliation should be discussed within a comprehensive multidisciplinary palliative care plan to achieve the best outcomes and maximize patient satisfaction. Surgical palliative care education should be an integral part of the surgical residency curricula and requires the development of specific competency assessment tools. The examination of the ethical principles involved in end-of life-care can help physicians in caring for their patients in the palliative care setting. In a multicultural society where individual freedoms are paramount, there are often no "right answers" when addressing bioethical dilemmas. However, a basic understanding of bioethical principles can aid physicians in navigating difficult decisions, for as a bioethicist once articulated, "the patient's stake in the matter is not always as clearly envisioned as it might be."[39]

REFERENCES

1. Dunn GP. The surgeon and palliative care: an evolving perspective. Surg Oncol Clin N Am 2001;10(1):7–24.
2. Dunn GP. Restoring palliative care as a surgical tradition. Bull Am Coll Surg 2004; 89(4):23–9.
3. National Quality Forum. A national framework and preferred practices for palliative care and hospice quality: a consensus report. 2006. Available at: www. qualityforum.org. Accessed August 11, 2010.
4. Easson AM, Crosby JA, Librach SL. Discussion of death and dying in surgical textbooks. Am J Surg 2001;182:34–9.
5. Bradley CT, Brasel KJ. Core competencies in palliative care for surgeons: interpersonal and communication skills. Am J Hosp Palliat Care 2008;24(6):499–507.
6. Surgeons Palliative Care Workgroup. Office of promoting excellence in end-of-life care: surgeon's palliative care workgroup report from the field. J Am Coll Surg 2003;197(4):661–86.
7. Galante JM, Bowles TL, Khatri VP, et al. Experience and attitudes of surgeons toward palliation in cancer. Arch Surg 2005;140(9):873–80.
8. Brasel KJ, Weissman DE. Palliative care education for surgeons. J Am Coll Surg 2004;199(3):495–9.
9. Weissman DE, Ambuel B, von Gunten CF, et al. Outcomes from a national multispecialty palliative care curriculum development project. J Palliat Med 2007; 10(2):408–19.

10. Klaristenfeld DD, Harrington DT, Miner TJ. Teaching palliative care and end-of-life issues: a core curriculum for surgical residents. Ann Surg Oncol 2007;14(6):1801–6.
11. Ross DD, Shpritz D, Alexander CS, et al. Development of required postgraduate palliative care training for internal medicine residents and medical oncology fellows. J Cancer Educ 2004;19:81–7.
12. Available at: http://134.192.120.12/canRes/htdocs/login.asp. Accessed August 17, 2010.
13. Available at: http://palliativecaretraining.org. Accessed August 17, 2010.
14. Chochinov HM. Dying, dignity and new horizons in palliative end-of-life care. CA Cancer J Clin 2006;56(2):84–109.
15. Chochinov HM. Dignity and the essence of medicine: the A, B, C, and D of dignity conserving care. BMJ 2007;335(7612):184–7.
16. Wagman LD. Progress in palliative surgery- is it a subspecialty? J Surg Oncol 2007;96:449–50.
17. Campbell ML. When will "usual care" in advanced illness be "palliative care"? J Palliat Med 2010;13(8):934–5.
18. Chipman JG, Beilman GJ, Schmitz CC, et al. Development and pilot testing of an OSCE for difficult conversations in surgical intensive care. J Surg Educ 2007; 64(2):79–87.
19. Helyer LK, O'Brien C, Coburn NG, et al. Surgeons' knowledge of quality indicators for gastric cancer surgery. Gastric Cancer 2007;10:205–14.
20. Forbes JF. Principles and potential of palliative surgery in patients with advanced cancer. Recent Results Cancer Res 1988;108:134–42.
21. Miner TJ, Jaques DP, Shriver C. Decision making on surgical palliation based on patient outcome data. Am J Surg 1999;177:150–4.
22. McCahill LE, Krouse R, Chu D, et al. Indications and use of palliative surgery-results of society of surgical oncology survey. Ann Surg Oncol 2002;9(1):104–12.
23. Blazeby JM. Measurement of outcome. Surg Oncol 2001;10:127–33.
24. McCahill LE, Krouse RS, Chu DZ, et al. Decision making in palliative surgery. J Am Coll Surg 2002;195(3):411–22 [discussion: 422–3].
25. Pellegrino ED. Is truth telling to the patient a cultural artifact? JAMA 1992;268(13): 1734–5.
26. Novack DH, Plumer R, Smith RL, et al. Changes in physicians' attitudes toward telling the cancer patient. JAMA 1979;241(9):897–900.
27. Annas GJ. Informed consent, cancer, and truth in prognosis. N Engl J Med 1994; 330(3):223–5.
28. Baile WF, Buckman R, Lenzi R, et al. SPIKES-A six-step protocol for delivering bad news: application to the patient with cancer. Oncologist 2000;5(4):302–11.
29. Dufault K, Martocchio BC. Symposium on compassionate care and the dying experience. Hope: its spheres and dimensions. Nurs Clin North Am 1985;20(2): 379–91.
30. Hedland S. Hope and communication in cancer care: what patients tell us. In: Angelos P, editor. Ethical issues in cancer patient care. New York: Springer; 2009. p. 65–77.
31. Gawande A. Letting go. The New Yorker. New York (NY): Conde Nast Publications; 2010.
32. Silveira MJ, Kim SY, Langa KM. Advance directives and outcomes of surrogate decision making before death. N Engl J Med 2010;362(13):1211–8.
33. Asch DA, Christakis NA. Why do physicians prefer to withdraw some forms of life support over others? Intrinsic attributes of life-sustaining treatments are associated with physicians' preferences. Med Care 1996;34(2):103–11.

34. Reynolds S, Cooper AB, McKneally M. Withdrawing life-sustaining treatment: ethical considerations. Surg Clin North Am 2007;87(4):919–36, viii.
35. Beauchamp TL, Childress JF. Principles of biomedical ethics. 6th edition. New York: Oxford University Press; 2009.
36. Hinshaw DB, Pawlik T, Mosenthal AC, et al. When do we stop, and how do we do it? Medical futility and withdrawal of care. J Am Coll Surg 2003;196(4):621–51.
37. Jonsen AR, Siegler M, Winsalde WJ. Clinical ethics. 6th edition. New York: McGraw-Hill Companies; 2006.
38. Grossman E, Angelos P. Futility: what Cool Hand Luke can teach the surgical community. World J Surg 2009;33(7):1338–40.
39. Sperry WL. The ethical basis of medical practice. New York: Paul B. Hoeber Inc; 1952.

Communication Skills in Palliative Surgery: Skill and Effort Are Key

Thomas J. Miner, MD

KEYWORDS

• Surgical palliation • Palliative triangle • Communication skills

The skill and effort that we put into our clinical communication does make an indelible impression on our patients, their families, and their friends. If we do it badly, they may never forgive us; if we do it well, they may never forget us.
— *Robert Buckman[1]*

Surgeons, by necessity, manage a broad spectrum of death and dying. Death can occur unexpectedly in the otherwise healthy individual because of an unexpected trauma, an unidentified medical condition, such as a ruptured aortic aneurysm, or a catastrophic perioperative event. A patient with severe burns or multiple organ failure in the intensive care unit may die after a period of prolonged uncertainty about possible recovery. Patients with chronic disease also die quite expectedly. Surgeons commonly care for and operate on such patients. Given the nature of their practice, surgeons require a broad expertise in communicating with patients and their families about these difficult circumstances.

The public and those in the medical profession are increasingly concerned about the adequacy and suitability of end-of-life care. Therapy aimed at prolonging life with little attention to relieving patient suffering has resulted in an increasing demand for placing quality of life over quantity of life. Government involvement and public discussions of death and dying often include debates about euthanasia and physician-assisted suicide, a move toward advance directives, and the need for improved hospice care.[2–5] Although comprehensive end-of-life care has been identified as the standard of care for dying patients, this care is widely recognized to be deficient.[6,7] Recent initiatives in palliative medicine, the therapeutic goals of which emphasize support and symptom management, are attempting to improve this critical aspect of the total care of patients with cancer.

Department of Surgery, The Alpert Medical School of Brown University, Rhode Island Hospital, 593 Eddy Street, APC 4, Providence, RI 02903, USA
E-mail address: TMiner@USASURG.org

Surg Clin N Am 91 (2011) 355–366
doi:10.1016/j.suc.2010.12.005
0039-6109/11/$ – see front matter © 2011 Elsevier Inc. All rights reserved.

surgical.theclinics.com

Being in twenty-first century, we confront a timeless and inescapable certainty of the human condition: that death is a natural fact of life.[8] About 50 years ago, it was common for physicians, patients, and families to avoid discussing cancer diagnoses. Conversations regarding diagnoses, treatment options, and prognoses, now take place routinely, and open disclosure has become a core principal of good clinical practice.[9] However, appropriate communication between patients and physicians is still lacking. In a recent study, more than 20% of patients were told their cancer diagnosis in an impersonal manner, suggesting that many physicians are either unacquainted with or unskilled at good communication. In a significant number of patients this communication in an impersonal manner was associated with a lack of trust or a bad relationship with the physician and was cited as a reason for changing physicians.[9] The high expectations of the general public and patients demand an effective use of communication skills to permit active participation in their health care decisions. At the end of life, patients and families seek well-developed communication and interpersonal skills to guide them during this particularly vulnerable time.[10]

SURGICAL PALLIATION

For decades, surgeons have been at the forefront in the movement toward palliative care. The roots of many current operations and operations used until recently to achieve a surgical "cure" can be traced back to procedures designed to alleviate symptomatic and often painful disease. In 1882, William Halstead introduced radical mastectomy to manage the pain emanating from locally advanced and ulcerating breast cancer, but this procedure was also found to be effective in sometimes curing cancer.[11] Similarly, coronary artery bypass grafting was first advocated for the symptomatic relief of angina pectoris but was then found to have survival benefits.[12] Many surgeons are not prepared to effectively administer palliative care despite a clear and well-established role. Surgical training in palliation is cursory, there is not enough quantity and quality of peer-reviewed literature,[4] and surgical textbooks[13] are generally lacking. This shortage of training and literature might explain why surgeons traditionally have been poor at communicating with patients about end-of-life issues.[14]

Palliative care has been defined by the World Health Organization[15] as "the total active care of patients whose disease is not responsive to curative treatment. Control of pain, of other symptoms, and of psychological, social, and spiritual problems, is paramount. The goal of palliative care is achievement of the best quality of life for patients and their families." Others have further defined surgical palliation to include (1) initial evaluation of the disease, (2) local control of the disease, (3) control of discharge or hemorrhage, (4) control of pain, and (5) reconstruction and rehabilitation. Although these broad definitions provide a global understanding of the reaches of palliative care, alternate interpretations of what constitutes a palliative surgical procedure by different clinicians and investigators render comparisons between and, at times, within studies problematic. Because ideal palliative care requires an approach defined in terms of the patient's individual needs and values, identical procedures may play dramatically different roles for each patient. Identifying surgical palliation by the type of procedure performed, rather than by the goals and intentions of the procedure, is of limited value. Designation of procedures as palliative based on the extent of disease (ranging from gross disease at operation to postoperative margin status) rather than on a sound understanding of the elements associated with good palliative therapy is equally fruitless. Surgical palliation is best defined as the deliberate use of a procedure in a patient with incurable disease with the intention of relieving symptoms, minimizing patient distress, and improving quality of life. Palliation is not the opposite of cure. Each term has its own distinct indications and goals that should be evaluated independently. By defining palliation based on factors such as symptom control and surgical intent, the primary focus on an individualized approach for palliative surgery is maintained. An association between palliative intent and surgical outcomes has been well demonstrated in patients with cancer in the literature. The effectiveness of a palliative intervention should be judged by the presence and durability of patient-acknowledged symptom resolution. During the palliative phase of care, endeavors to improve the overall survival should not outweigh the efforts aimed at minimizing the morbidity, mortality, or duration of treatment. Although symptom palliation may result in increased survival for the individual patient, it is inappropriate to select a palliative procedure based solely on a desire for improved duration of survival.[16–20]

Palliation of complications from advanced cancer demands the highest level of surgical judgment and serves as an excellent model for considering surgical palliation. Although surgical issues for cancer sites can differ, the indications for surgical palliative procedures generally fall into 3 main areas of concern: obstruction, bleeding, and perforation. Individual patients also may present with more chronic complaints such as pain, nausea, vomiting, inability to eat, anemia, or jaundice. When considering the appropriate and effective use of palliative procedures, a surgeon is often confronted with a full range of multidisciplinary treatment options and technical considerations that could potentially relieve some of the symptoms of an advanced malignancy. Practitioners must often deliberate over options that are outside their individual experience. Although consideration of risk in terms of treatment-related toxicity, morbidity, and mortality is an important part of the surgical decision-making process, attention to this element should not be the sole factor in making decisions about palliative therapy. Decisions are best made on end points such as the probability of symptom resolution, the effect on overall quality of life, pain control, and cost effectiveness. Regardless of the anatomic site and cause leading to the need for palliative intervention, deliberations over surgical palliation must consider the medical condition and performance status of the patient, the natural history of the primary and secondary symptoms, the extent and prognosis of the cancer, the potential success and durability of the procedure, the availability and success of nonsurgical management, and the individual patient's quality and expectancy of life. Owing to the significant morbidity and mortality associated with palliative procedures, the single most important factor demonstrated in the literature in successful palliation is clearly proper patient selection. Because of the limited research and predominately anecdotal experience in this field, treatment algorithms and well-established surgical dictums are essentially nonexistent. However, from the largest prospective trial to date, it is known that poor performance status, poor nutrition, and no previous cancer therapy are factors that indicate patients who will do poorly.[20] Through the palliative phase of a patient's disease, specific complaints may change and goals may be redefined many times. Therapy for symptoms must remain flexible and individualized to meet continually the patient's unique and ever-changing needs. This is a situation in which surgical judgment is imperative, because these problems cannot be thought of in terms of right or wrong.[21]

Optimal palliative decision making is facilitated through effective interactions and direct communication between the patient, family members, and the surgeon through an indomitable relationship described as palliative triangle (**Fig. 1**). Through the dynamics of the triangle, the patient's complaints, values, and emotional support are considered against the known medical and surgical alternatives. Outcomes data

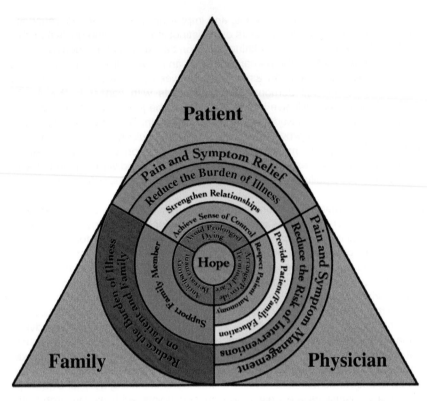

Palliation Triangle

Fig. 1. The palliative triangle. Interactions between the patient, the family, and the surgeon guide individual decisions regarding palliative care. The hope for potentially achievable goals is advanced as each participant of the palliative triangle fulfills specific obligations. Good communication between the patient, the family, and the surgeon is essential for the palliative triangle to be effective. (*From* Thomay AA, Jaques DP, Miner TJ. Surgical palliation: getting back to our roots. Surg Clin North Am 2009;89:33; with permission.)

obtained through reports on surgical palliation can be especially useful to submit accurate information regarding chance of success, procedure-related durability, the possibility for complications, and anticipated survival. Another important factor is anticipating, understanding, and addressing a patient's and/or a family's expectations about the intent of the proposed procedure. The palliative intent needs to be understood and explicitly agreed upon. Although patients, family members, and surgeons may at times have incongruent expectations, the dynamics of the palliative triangle help to moderate such beliefs and guide the decision-making process toward the best possible choice for the patient. This strong relationship may also explain the observation of high patient satisfaction toward surgeons after palliative operations, even in patients having no demonstrable benefit from surgery or in those experiencing serious complications. Patients are satisfied because the surgeon was there for them at this difficult time of great need; discussed the risks, benefits, and alternatives of all of their choices; and remained engaged with them throughout the remainder of their lives.[14,16]

Even though the thoughtfulness, judgment, and time required to make such complicated palliative decisions are appreciated by patients and families, some physicians and surgeons shy away from this process with the explanation that they do not want to take away hope from those battling cancer. Cleary, it is inappropriate to suggestprolonged survival to be provided by an operation performed with a palliative intent. Rather than focusing on what cannot be provided (cure), emphasis must be placed on those things that can be realistically delivered. As the palliative triangle suggests, a successful palliative surgeon places this definition of hope at the center of a patient's overall care. It is rational for the patient with advanced cancer to hope for quality of life, symptom resolution, technically superior palliative operations, dignity, and compassion. Through continued personal interactions and deliberate communication, each participant of the palliative triangle contributes to making a unique patient-centered decision, recognizing that varying procedures will have different goals for every individual. Although identical procedures can be performed for similar clinical problems, whether it is right of wrong depends on the unique circumstances of each patient.[14]

The discipline has evolved to recognize that palliative surgical treatment options are not right for every patient and that care must be individualized in a multidisciplinary manner that is most appropriate for a specific patient. There will be times when the most appropriate decision a surgeon can make in the treatment of a terminally ill patient is not to perform an operation. However, this means that a surgeon will have to say "no" to a significant number of patients, who are thought to possess too much risk without a reasonable expectation of benefit. Surgeons must be cautious never to promise an outcome that they cannot realistically expect to deliver. When recognizing those patients who are at risk for procedure-related complications or death or those in whom a particular procedure is unlikely to provide an idealized benefit, surgeons should understand that saying "no" is appropriate. If communicated effectively, the patient will ultimately understand that this response does not represent abandonment or failure on the part of the surgeon but rather a team approach to minimizing symptoms without sacrificing quality of life.[14]

SURGEONS AS COMMUNICATORS

Effective use of communication skills by physicians benefits both the physician and the patient and is a key element of a successful therapeutic relationship. Physicians' communication skills are associated with important patient and physician outcomes.[22,23] These outcomes include physician and patient satisfaction,[24,25] patient participation in care and adjustment to illness,[26] malpractice liability,[27] and important clinical markers of health.[28–31] When doctors communicate well with their patients, clinical problems are identified more accurately, patients are more satisfied with their care, treatment plans are more likely to be followed, feelings of distress and vulnerability are lessened, and physicians' well-being is improved.[32] Back and colleagues[33] argue that although physicians often learn good interviewing skills, their training does not promote proficiency in second-order communication skills, such as conveying empathy and understanding. This lack of training complicates situations in which bad or difficult news is commonly discussed. Some find that their lack of training or discomfort with emotionally charged negative information at times leads to unpleasant interactions.[34]

The importance of good communication skills in surgical practice is undeniable.[10] One study comparing primary care physicians with surgeons showed that surgeons spend more time emphasizing patient education and counseling.[35] Surgeons deliver bad news frequently in the course of their careers.[36] Surgeons are confronted, not uncommonly, with other challenging experiences such as requesting permission for autopsy or organ donation.[23] Because surgeons frequently deal with gravely sick and dying patients, surveyed surgeons have identified breaking bad news and bereavement counseling as areas worthy of instruction for surgical trainees.[37]

Surgical competence in palliative care requires not only sound clinical decision making but also skill in communication and building relationships. Although communication barriers may involve the patient and family, or even the health system itself, the surgeon bears the major responsibility for conducting the communications well.[38] Communication is often the most important component of palliative care, and effective symptom control is virtually impossible without effective communication.[39] In addition to the fact that communication provides the structure and context of good surgical palliative decisions, it is sometimes all that can be offered. Compared with other palliative therapies, communication skills have clear palliative efficacy (reduces patient anxiety and distress) and a wide therapeutic index (treatment-related morbidity and mortality is rare), and their most common problem in practice is suboptimal dosing.[1]

Most surgeons are not trained in effective communication techniques and are left to learn by trial and error and frequently miss empathic opportunities.[40] Although some surgeons through practice, intuition, or study are highly skilled at delivering bad news and at negotiating patients' reactions to bad news empathically, many are not as effective communicators as they think they are or should be.[34] An effort to improve surgical palliative care in the future will require the thoughtful education of future and current surgeons not only in sound palliative decision making but also in communication skills. With the restrictions to residency training secondary to managed care and work hour regulations, surgical training programs have increasingly become algorithm based. Although this transformation likely works with the old surgical adage of "see one, do one, teach one," all too often, residents looking for guidance in the proper conversations of palliative care never get the opportunity to "see one." Robert Milch summed up this idea best in his talk on palliative care in surgical resident education at the American College of Surgeons Clinical Congress in 2003 as, "if you think about it, demonstration of competency in communication skills is much like performing an operation. We would never think of sending an untutored, un-mentored, unsupervised house officer into an operating room to do a procedure never seen, modeled, or performed before, and about which he had only read in a book. Yet this sort of demand for communication skills is one on which we place our house officers all the time, and they have not been taught good communication skills. And very often they have not seen it modeled or mentored."[41]

Although there are several programs to improve communication skills in surgical trainees, the vast majority of surgical training programs have no set curriculum in which to teach palliative care.[34,42,43] However, in a study from the author's institution, 47 general surgery residents were surveyed, and all thought that managing end-of life issues are valuable skills for a surgeon and that sessions in this topic would be a useful and important part of their training. The study was based on a pilot curriculum in palliative surgical care designed specifically for residents. The curriculum was presented over three 1-hour sessions, and included didactic sessions, group discussions, and role-playing scenarios, and the residents were asked to complete pretest, posttest, and 3-month follow-up surveys. Specific modules to improve communication skill and breaking bad news were included in the workshop. At pretest, only 9% of the residents thought that they had previously received adequate training in palliation during their residency and only 57% stated that they felt comfortable speaking to patients about end-of-life issues. At posttest and 3-month follow-up, however, these goals were met for 85% of the residents. Although this study was not designed for mastery of this complex topic, it demonstrated that surgeons can be introduced effectively to palliative care early in their careers with only a modest time commitment. Residents cited that their biggest problem in interacting with patient and families regarding end-of-life issues was apprehension about dealing with extreme emotional responses. Learning communication techniques to help them navigate effectively through these difficult situations seemed to help trainees overcome this barrier.[44] When used correctly, lessons such as these in conversation and advanced decision making can provide the building block to successful palliation spanning an entire career.[45] Because many efforts such as these to improve communication skills focus on medical students and residents, they often remain isolated in academic settings. The communication skills of the busy surgeon often remain poorly developed, and the need for established physicians to become better communicators continues.[34]

IMPROVING COMMUNICATION SKILLS

In the 1970s and 1980s, it was widely assumed that communication skills were an innate ability. Coupled with a belief that practitioners should be able to feel or sense what the patient experiences in order to respond intuitively in an appropriate way, many doctors felt alienated to the topic of patient-physician communication because it was excessively "touch-feely." Such a paradigm offers few suggestions or guidelines that could help even highly motivated physicians to improve their skills. In the last 2 to 3 decades, however, researchers have learned that communications skills are acquired skills like any other clinical ability and are not some intangible inherited gift. The knowledge, skills, and behaviors associated with effective communication can be learned and retained with a few techniques applied in a logical sequence.[38,39]

Although there are probably many ways of summarizing and simplifying medical communication, the most practical and popular technique is the context, listening, acknowledgement, strategy, and summary (CLASS) protocol of Buckman.[39] This 5-step basic protocol for medical communication, bearing the acronym CLASS, is easy to remember and use. It also lays a straightforward method for dealing with emotions. The ability to empathize with patients is fundamental to the ultimate success of the exchange but is frequently undervalued because of the disproportionate importance that is placed on reasoning capacity in medical care. As summarized in **Fig. 2**, the CLASS protocol identifies the following 5 main components of medical communication as essential and crucial: context (the physical context or setting), listening skills, acknowledgement of patient's emotions, strategy for clinical management, and summary.[38,39]

The ability to discuss bad news with the patient and family is a clinical skill that is essential for effective communication during end-of-life care. Bad news can be defined as any news that adversely affects patients' view of their future. The goal of skillfully breaking bad news is to reduce the severity and duration of stress and encourage engagement of coping mechanisms, both for physicians and for patients and their caregivers. Learning skills to improve breaking bad news can help to prevent potentially devastating physician interactions leading to the insensitively blunt delivery or "dumping" of bad news to patients and their families. Such occurrences of the "hit and run" delivery of bad news likely result from physicians' own emotional discomfort, perceived lack of time, and insufficient training in empathic communication skills.[34] The setting, patient's perception, invitation, knowledge, emotions, and strategy/summary (SPIKES) protocol (**Fig. 3**), a variant of the basic CLASS approach, has

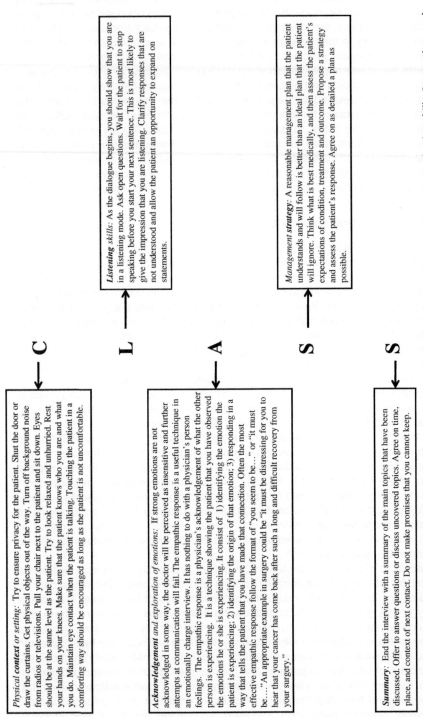

Fig. 2. The CLASS protocol. It is a basic method that can be used by any health care professional in improving communication skills. Suggestions on how to implement each element of the protocol are offered. (*Adapted from* Buckman R. Communication skills in palliative care: a practical guide. Neurol Clin 2001;19:989–1004; with permission.)

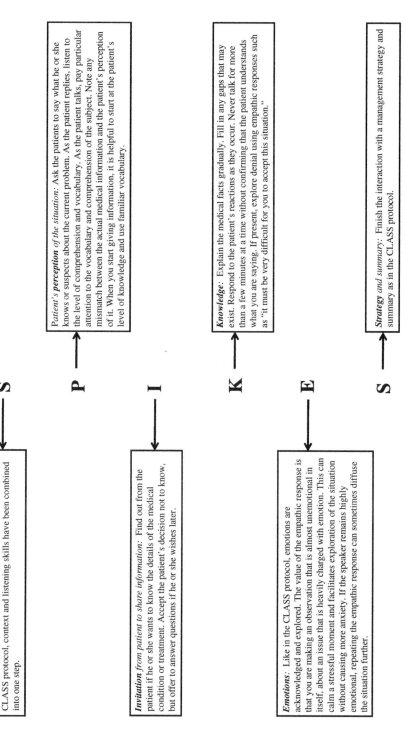

S

Setting (context and listing skills): The first two steps of the CLASS protocol, context and listening skills have been combined into one step.

P

*Patient's **perception** of the situation:* Ask the patients to say what he or she knows or suspects about the current problem. As the patient replies, listen to the level of comprehension and vocabulary. As the patient talks, pay particular attention to the vocabulary and comprehension of the subject. Note any mismatch between the actual medical information and the patient's perception of it. When you start giving information, it is helpful to start at the patient's level of knowledge and use familiar vocabulary.

I

Invitation from patient to share information: Find out from the patient if he or she wants to know the details of the medical condition or treatment. Accept the patient's decision not to know, but offer to answer questions if he or she wishes later.

K

Knowledge: Explain the medical facts gradually. Fill in any gaps that may exist. Respond to the patient's reactions as they occur. Never talk for more than a few minutes at a time without confirming that the patient understands what you are saying. If present, explore denial using empathic responses such as "it must be very difficult for you to accept this situation."

E

Emotions: Like in the CLASS protocol, emotions are acknowledged and explored. The value of the empathic response is that you are making an observation that is almost unemotional in itself, about an issue that is heavily charged with emotion. This can calm a stressful moment and facilitates exploration of the situation without causing more anxiety. If the speaker remains highly emotional, repeating the empathic response can sometimes diffuse the situation further.

S

Strategy and summary: Finish the interaction with a management strategy and summary as in the CLASS protocol.

Fig. 3. The SPIKES protocol. The listed steps offer a helpful systematic approach of communicating at times when stress is high, such as when delivering bad news. Suggestions on how to implement each element of the protocol are offered. (*Adapted from* Buckman R. Communication skills in palliative care: a practical guide. Neurol Clin 2001;19:989–1004; with permission.)

been designed specifically for the purpose of successfully communicating bad news with patients and families.[39]

SUMMARY

The ability to effectively communicate with patients and families is a clinical skill that is essential for effective end-of-life care. Good communication about symptom severity, patient preferences, and patient expectations can help the physician make useful and relevant clinical decisions that can be shared with patients and their families. Forthright and compassionate discussions about terminal disease, including prognosis and treatment options, further allow patients and families to prepare for the final stages of life. Good communication can help providers, families, and patients to "clarify and achieve their hopes and goals within the constraints of progressive disease."[46] Using well-defined communication tools and systematic approach can facilitate this challenging task.

Incorporating communication skills to provide excellent surgical palliative care into surgical practice takes time, effort, experience, understanding, and compassion. Obtaining these skills requires only time and a desire to improve on the care given by surgeons to their patients with the same commitment that is routinely given to a new technical procedure or treatment plan.

REFERENCES

1. Buckman R. Communications and emotions: skills and effort are key. BMJ 2002; 325:672.
2. Singer PA, Martin DK, Kelner M. Quality end-of-life care: patient perspectives. JAMA 1999;281:163–8.
3. Steinhauser KE, Christakis NA, Clipp EC, et al. Factors considered important at the end of life by patients, family, physicians, and other care providers. JAMA 2000;284:2476–82.
4. Miner TJ, Tavaf-Motamen H, Shriver CD, et al. An evaluation of surgical palliation based on patient outcome data. Am J Surg 1999;177:150–4.
5. Hampson LA, Emanuel EJ. The prognosis for changes in end-of-life care after the Schiavo case. Health Aff (Millwood) 2005;24:972–5.
6. Lynn J. Learning of care for people with chronic illness facing the end of life. JAMA 2000;284:2508–11.
7. A controlled trial to improve care for seriously ill hospitalized patients. The study to understand prognoses and preferences for outcomes and risks of treatments (SUPPORT). The SUPPORT principal investigators. JAMA 2000;274:1591–8.
8. McCue JD. The naturalness of dying. JAMA 1995;273:1039–43.
9. Figg WD, Smith EK, Price DK, et al. Disclosing a diagnosis of cancer: where and how does it occur? J Clin Oncol 2010;28:3630–5.
10. Bradley CT, Brasel KJ. Core competencies in palliative care for surgeons: interpersonal and communications skills. Am J Hosp Pall Med 2008;24:299–507.
11. Halstead WJ. The results of radical operations for the cure of cancer of the breast. Ann Surg 1907;46:1–27.
12. McCahill LE, Dunn GP, Mosenthal AC, et al. Palliation as a core surgical principle: part 1. J Am Coll Surg 2004;199(1):149–60.
13. Easson AM, Crosby JA, Librach SL. Discussion of death and dying in surgical textbooks. Am J Surg 2001;182:34–9.
14. Thomay AA, Jaques DP, Miner TJ. Surgical palliation: getting back to our roots. Surg Clin North Am 2009;89:27–41.

15. World Health Organization. Cancer pain relief and palliative cure: report of a WHO expert committee (technical report series No. 804). Geneva (Switzerland): World Health Organization; 1990. p. 11.
16. Miner TJ, Jaques DP, Shriver CD. A prospective evaluation of patients undergoing surgery for the palliation of an advanced malignancy. Ann Surg Oncol 2002;9:696–703.
17. Miner TJ, Jaques DP, Paty P, et al. Symptom control of locally recurrent rectal cancer. Ann Surg Oncol 2002;10:72–9.
18. Miner TJ, Jaques DP, Karpeh MS, et al. Defining non-curative gastric resections by palliative intent. J Am Coll Surg 2004;198:1013–21.
19. Miner TJ, Karpeh MS. Gastrectomy for gastric cancer: defining critical elements of patient selection and outcome assessment. Surg Oncol Clin N Am 2004;13: 455–66.
20. Miner TJ, Brennan MF, Jaques DP. A prospective, symptom related, outcomes analysis of 1,022 palliative procedures for advanced cancer. Ann Surg 2004; 240:719–27.
21. Miner TJ. Palliative surgery for advanced cancer: lessons learned in patient selection and outcome assessment. Am J Clin Oncol 2005;28:411–4.
22. Makoul G. Essential elements of communication in medical encounters: the Kalamazoo consensus statement. Acad Med 2001;76:390–3.
23. Kalet AL, Janicik R, Schwarz M, et al. Teaching communication skills on the surgery clerkship. Med Educ Online 2005;10:1–7.
24. Levinson W, Stiles WB, Inui TS, et al. Physician frustration in communicating with patients. Med Care 1993;31:285–95.
25. McLafferty RB, Williams RG, Lambert AD, et al. Surgeon communication behaviors that lead patients to not recommend the surgeon to family members or friends: analysis and impact. Surgery 2006;140:616–24.
26. Eisenthal S, Koopman C, Stoeckle JD. The nature of patients' requests for physicians' help. Acad Med 1990;65:401–5.
27. Levinson W, Roter DL, Mullooly JP, et al. Physician patient communication: the relationship with malpractice claims among primary care physicians and surgeons. JAMA 1997;277:553–9.
28. Kaplan SH, Greenfield S, Ware JE. Assessing the effects of physician-patient interactions on the outcomes of chronic disease. Med Care 1989;27: S110–27.
29. Rost KM, Flavin KS, Cole K, et al. Change in metabolic control and functional status after hospitalization. Diabetes Care 1991;14:881–9.
30. Mumfor K, Schlesinger HJ, Glass GV. The effect of psychological intervention on recovery from surgery and heart attacks: an analysis of the literature. Am J Public Health 1982;72:141–51.
31. Fallowfield LJ, Hall A, Maguire GP, et al. Psychological outcomes of different treatment policies in women with early breast cancer outside a clinical trial. BMJ 1990;301:575–80.
32. Maguire P, Pitceathly C. Key communication skills and how to acquire them. BMJ 2002;325:697700.
33. Back AL, Arnold RM, Baile WF, et al. Approaching difficult communication tasks in oncology. CA Cancer J Clin 2005;55:164–77.
34. Helft PR, Petronio S. Communication pitfalls with cancer patients: "hit-and-run" deliveries of bad news. J Am Coll Surg 2007;205:807–11.
35. Levinson W, Chaumeton N. Communication between surgeons and patients in routine office visits. Surgery 1999;125:127–34.

36. Eggly S, Penner LA, Albrecht TL, et al. Discussing bad news in the outpatient oncology clinic: rethinking current communication guidelines. J Clin Oncol 2006;24(4):716–9.

37. Sise MJ, Sise CB, Sack DI, et al. Surgeons' attitudes about communicating with patients and their families. Curr Surg 2006;63:213–8.

38. Milch RA, Dunn GP. Communication: part of the surgical armamentarium. J Am Coll Surg 2001;193:449–51.

39. Buckman R. Communication skills in palliative care: a practical guide. Neurol Clin 2001;19:989–1004.

40. Easter DW, Beach W. Competent patient care is dependent upon attending to empathetic opportunities presented during interview sessions. Curr Surg 2004; 61:313–8.

41. McCahill LE, Dunn GP, Mosenthal AC, et al. Palliation as a core surgical principle: part 2. J Am Coll Surg 2004;199(2):321–34.

42. Von Gunten CF, Ferris FD, Emanuel LL. Ensuring competency in end-of-life care: communication and relational skills. JAMA 2000;284:3051–7.

43. Traveline JM, Ruchinskas R, D'Alonzo GE. Patient-physician communication: why and how. J Am Osteopath Assoc 2005;105:13–8.

44. Klaristenfeld DD, Harrington DT, Miner TJ. Teaching palliative care and end-of-life issues: a core curriculum for surgical residents. Ann Surg Oncol 2007;14(6): 1801–6.

45. Huffman JL. Educating surgeons for the new golden hours: honing the skills of palliative care. Surg Clin North Am 2005;85(2):383–91.

46. Gordon G. Care not cure: dialogues at the transition. Patient Educ Couns 2003; 50:95–8.

Image-Guided Palliative Care Procedures

Jay Requarth, MD

KEYWORDS

- Cholecystostomy • Chemoembolization • Indwelling catheters
- Radiotherapy • Transjugular intrahepatic portasystemic shunt
- Palliation

Image-guided palliative procedures are often performed in interventional radiology.[1] The image-guided procedures discussed in this article are used to alleviate the pain and suffering of patients with malignancies and/or multiple comorbidities. It is not possible to discuss, in detail, the entire breadth of image-guided palliative procedures; thus, only a few of the more commonly requested procedures are reviewed (all are percutaneous): cholecystostomy, biliary decompression, enteral feeding and decompression tubes, chemical neurolysis (for pain control), cementoplasty, tunneled drainage catheters, transjugular intrahepatic portasystemic shunt, pleurodesis, tube thoracostomy, thermal and chemical tumor ablation, transcatheter arterial chemoembolization (TACE), and selective internal radiation therapy (SIRT). A decision tree is given with each procedure/disease to guide the discussion. Palliative urologic and thoracic procedures are discussed elsewhere in this issue.

Interventional radiologists are uniquely skilled as palliative care providers. As imagers, radiologists have extensive experience in diagnostic image interpretation and disease prognostication. Additionally, interventional radiologists have an array of both therapeutic and palliative interventions to offer patients coping with a life-threatening illness.[2] Although Samuel Shem's[3] sixth law in *The House of God* states that any body cavity can be reached with a 14-gauge needle and a good strong arm, interventional radiologists are expert at determining if a needle, tube, or probe can get there safely—strong arm or not.

Both surgeons and interventional radiologists need to understand that a patient's end-of-life goals can be challenging to elucidate and difficult to manage. When Medicare beneficiaries are faced with a hypothetical terminal illness, more Medicare beneficiaries were concerned about getting too much treatment than too little (45.0% vs 40.4%).[4] But patient preferences are a moving target, especially when faced with

The author has nothing to disclose.

Section of Vascular and Interventional Radiology, Department of Radiology, Wake Forest University Baptist Medical Center, Medical Center Boulevard, Winston Salem, NC 27157, USA

E-mail address: jrequart@wfubmc.edu

Surg Clin N Am 91 (2011) 367–402

doi:10.1016/j.suc.2010.12.009

0039-6109/11/$ – see front matter © 2011 Elsevier Inc. All rights reserved.

surgical.theclinics.com

real (as compared with theoretical) chronic diseases. Fried and colleagues[5] found that the acceptability of treatment burdens increases as patients experience a decline in their state of health. Whiteneck and colleagues[6] found that 64% of high-cervical quadriplegia patients who have been on a respirator for more than a year rated their quality of life as good or excellent. As summarized by Dr Thomas Finucane,[7] patients face death with a "deeply held desire not to be dead."

None of the palliative care treatments discussed in this article have been evaluated using comparative effectiveness research, despite the fact that the Institute of Medicine places "coordinated care...and usual care in long-term and end-of-life care of the elderly" in the second quartile of the top 100 initial national priority topics.[8] Even if the palliative treatments discussed in this article provide a statistically significant improvement in survival, the treatment may not be justified and/or reimbursed if the cost is greater than $50,000 to $100,000 per quality-adjusted life year.[9–11] Evaluating these palliative treatments against supportive care, operative treatments, and palliative chemotherapy is needed to fully integrate them into end-of-life patient management.[12,13]

TECHNIQUES IN INTERVENTIONAL RADIOLOGY

Vascular and interventional radiology is a difficult field to describe because rather than being organized around an organ system and/or disease, the field is organized around image-guided therapeutic techniques. Although surgeons may feel that these image-guided techniques are easily mastered, the American Board of Surgery and the American Board of Radiology have published a statement that acknowledges the need for specialized image interpretation training and the potential conflict between vascular surgeons and interventional radiologists. General and vascular surgeons are to use endovascular techniques to treat vascular disease, whereas interventional radiologists are to use endovascular techniques to treat end-organ disease and vascular disease.[14]

The interventional radiology procedures discussed in this article can be grouped into image catheter placement, purposeful endovascular arterial obstruction (embolotherapy), endovascular drug administration, endovascular delivery of radioactive particles, and percutaneous thermal or chemical ablation.

IMAGE-GUIDED CATHETER PLACEMENT

Image-guided catheter placement requires experience with 2-D B-mode ultrasound and fluoroscopy. Higher-frequency transducers give excellent images of superficial structures, but the image attenuation increases with depth. Lower-frequency transducers can be used to image deeper structures, but the image quality is, at times, challenging. Fluoroscopy is a skill easily mastered by surgeons, but patient and physician radiation safety is an often overlooked problem until radiation injury (to a patient and/or physician) is encountered. Surgeons interested in using fluoroscopy are encouraged to educate themselves on the basics of radiation physics and safety.

EMBOLOTHERAPY

Embolotherapy involves the endovascular delivery of vascular occlusion agents, such as chemical agents (absolute alcohol or 5% phenol), absorbable porcine gelatin sponge (Gelfoam, Pfizer, Pharmacia & Upjohn Co, New York, NY, USA), embolic particles, fibered metal coils, and cyanoacrylate glues. Often requiring the use of microcatheters with internal diameters of 0.025 in or smaller, embolotherapy can be used to stop hemorrhage in inoperable patients and to produce ischemia in tumors (**Fig. 1**). Although it can be used throughout the body, transcatheter arterial embolotherapy (with or without additional chemotherapy or radioactive particles) is particularly effective in the liver because hepatic tumors larger than 5 mm receive the vast majority of their blood supply from the hepatic artery, whereas normal liver cells receive most of their blood supply from the postal vein.[15] The tumor arteries range in size from 25 to 75 micrometers.

TRANSCATHETER ARTERIAL CHEMOEMBOLIZATION

TACE involves endovascular delivery of chemotherapy agent(s) and a free acyl-ethyl-ester emulsions, followed by embolic agents. Randomized controlled trials are lacking, but data suggest that there is improved survival with TACE over transcatheter arterial embolotherapy without chemotherapy.[16] Adding chemotherapeutic agents (such as cisplatin, doxorubicin, and mitomycin) to embolic agents results in tumor drug concentrations that are up to 2-fold higher than in nontumor hepatic cells and measurable drug levels that last for up to 1 month (**Figs. 2** and **3**).[17,18]

Most TACE regimens include Ethiodol (Guerbet LLC, Bloomington, IN, USA) as the ester emulsion, although no randomized controlled trials have been performed to justify its inclusion.[19] Mistakenly described as an oil in many publications,[20–22] Ethiodol is the ethyl ester of a hydrogenated fatty acid (possibly stearic acid) derived from poppy seed oil. Although the exact solution is a closely held corporate secret, it is described by the package insert as a 70:30 mixture of the ester with an unnamed diluent. Ethiodol acts as a radio-opaque agent that occludes microscopic arteries[17,21] and helps emulsify chemotherapy agents for infusion.[18–22]

SELECTIVE INTERNAL RADIATION THERAPY

Although liver tumors are sensitive to external beam radiotherapy, with tumoricidal doses starting at approximately 120 Gy, radiation doses larger than 30 Gy result in radiation hepatitis and liver failure. The arterial blood supply to tumorous and normal

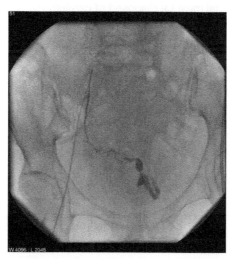

Fig. 1. Digital subtraction angiography of the anterior division of the right internal iliac artery in a woman with unresectable cervical cancer who developed significant vaginal bleeding. Embolotherapy using fibered metal coils controlled the hemorrhage.

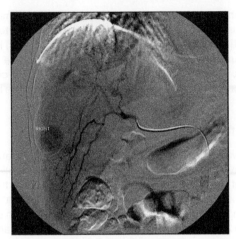

Fig. 2. Fluoroscopic image of TACE administered to segment 6 of the right lobe of the liver in a patient with HCC. The iodinated contrast is concentrated in the arterial vasculature of the HCC tumor reflecting the dense arterial network feeding the tumor.

liver is unique with a 3-fold increase in the number of arterial capillaries feeding tumors as feed normal liver; most of the blood supply to normal liver is from the portal veins.[23,24] SIRT was developed as a method of preferentially delivering high-dose radiation to liver tumors using these unique vascular findings. SIRT uses an embolic agent embedded with yttrium 90, which is a pure beta-emitting isotope (physical half-life of 64 hours) with mean and maximum penetrations of 2.5 mm and 10 mm, respectively.[25] Repeated doses of intra-arterial yttrium 90 microspheres can deliver a maximum cumulated dose of approximately 1600 Gy.[26] Evaluation of explanted livers found a 50% to 85% necrosis in hepatocellular carcinoma (HCC) tumors and a 90% necrosis in colorectal liver metastases (CRLM) tumors.[27] Yttrium 90–impregnated particles are extremely expensive and require specialized delivery systems. All contaminated material must be disposed of carefully.

Before the radioembolotherapy, angiography and scintographic lung shunt fraction must be assessed.[25] During angiography, the detailed anatomy of the celiac axis and

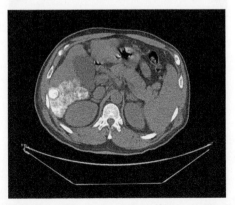

Fig. 3. Noncontrast axial image of the same patient shown in **Fig. 2**. The small peripheral HCC is densely opacified with Lipiodol because the viscous material occludes the small arteries of the tumor. This opacification will remain for several weeks to months.

superior mesenteric artery must be determined; the falciform, right or left inferior phrenic, inferior esophageal, right or accessory gastric, supra- and retroduodenal, and accessory right hepatic arteries may require prophylactic embolization. Lung scintigraphy with technetium 99m macroaggregated albumin scan showing pulmonary delivery of more than 30 Gy in one treatment is a contraindication to radioembolization because of the risk of radiation pneumonitis. Complications of radioembolization include postradioembolization syndrome (20%–55%), hepatic dysfunction (0%–4%), biliary injury (<10%), portal hypertension (rare), radiation pneumonitis (<1%), gastrointestinal ulceration (<5%), vascular injury, lymphopenia, and periumbilical pain. In the absence of off-target embolization complications, patients treated with yttrium 90 complain of fatigue (61%), nausea (21%), and vague abdominal pain (25%).[28]

LOCOREGIONAL THERAPY

Image-guided locoregional therapy consists of localized tumor destruction using chemical and thermal ablation (**Table 1**).[29–33] Both absolute alcohol (ethanol) and 5% to 10% phenol solutions are commonly used as chemical ablation agents. Thermal ablation uses either extreme heat or cold to kill tissue. Radiofrequency ablation (RFA) and microwave ablation are the most commonly used thermal ablative techniques (**Figs. 4** and **5**). Although many of these ablative techniques are unfamiliar to surgeons, radiofrequency energy has been used by surgeons for nearly a century in the form of the Bovie knife.[2] The use of locoregional treatment in oncology patients has been growing at a compounded annual growth rate of 22% since 2002.[33] Although open ablation procedures are seeing a flat to negative growth rate, image-guided ablation procedures are increasing significantly with more than 90% of all ablation procedures performed by radiologists. Nevertheless, urologists now perform 35% of all percutaneous cryoablation and 10% of all percutaneous RFA procedures.

CHOLECYSTOSTOMY FOR CHOLECYSTITIS

Cholecystitis is a common problem in the United States; more than 900,000 cholecystectomies are performed yearly (**Fig. 6**).[34,35] Major in-hospital complications identified after laparoscopic cholecystectomy are associated with comorbidities rather than surgeon or hospital operative volumes.[36] Performing, or conversion to, an open cholecystectomy is associated with advanced age and a high comorbidity burden.[37] When compared with laparoscopic cholecystectomy, open cholecystectomy is associated with a higher overall morbidity (17.7% vs 3.1%), serious morbidity (11.1% vs 1.4%), and mortality (2.8% vs 0.3%). In addition to the increased morbidity and mortality associated with open cholecystectomy, many of these patients are treated medically, then discharged without surgical treatment of their cholelithiasis/cholecystitis. Using a Medicare database, Riall and colleagues[38] found that 25% of Medicare beneficiaries admitted for acute cholecystitis during the decade ending in 2005 did not undergo cholecystectomy during the index admission; presumably, some of those patients had high comorbidity burdens. The resulting cost to the health care system, and morbidity to patients, was significant because 38% of the surviving patients not treated with cholecystectomy were readmitted with recurrent cholecystitis or gallstone-related diseases, such as pancreatitis.

Considering this information, emergency cholecystectomy should be a procedure of historical significance only. High-risk patients need to have their sepsis controlled before surgery; furthermore, the surgery needs to be performed in the light of day with optimal support for surgeons. In addition, patients should not be considered

Table 1
Locoregional ablative therapies

Percutaneous Ablation Technique	Energy Conduction	Cell Death Mechanism	Visualize Ablation Zone?	Ablation Zone Pain?	Use Multiple Probes Simultaneously?	Thermal Sink Issues?	Bleeding Problems?
RFA	Electrical circuit	Coagulation necrosis	Yes	Yes	No	Yes	No
Microwave	Dielectric-hysteresis	Coagulation necrosis	Yes	Yes	Yes (exponential effect)	Yes	No
Cryotherapy	Thermal (rapid cooling)	Intra- and extracellular freezing	Yes[a]	No	Yes	Yes	Yes
PEA	Chemical	Desiccation	No	Yes	No	No	No

Abbreviation: PEA, percutaneous ethanol ablation.
[a] Excellent visualization—best of the thermal ablation techniques.

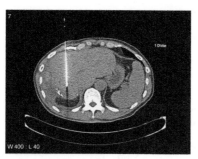

Fig. 4. Noncontrast axial CT during RFA treatment of recurrent CRLM years after right hepatic segmentectomy. For tumors larger than 3 cm in diameter, multiple treatments are necessary.

too ill for treatment of symptomatic cholelithiasis. Much like the treatment of an abscess, percutaneous cholecystostomy is an effective treatment for patients with cholecystitis. Described by Radder[39] in 1980, a percutaneous drainage catheter can be placed with local anesthesia using 2-D B-mode ultrasound, with or without fluoroscopy, with excellent results.[39–46] The major complication, bile leakage, is rare (approximately 3%).[42] Cholecystostomy will not treat cholangitis if the cystic duct is occluded; thus, additional procedures may be necessary.

PALLIATIVE BILIARY DECOMPRESSION

Obstructive jaundice is associated with pruritus, sepsis, liver dysfunction, and malnutrition; if untreated, life expectancy is short and death is uncomfortable (**Figs. 7–9**). Surgical drainage using a segment 3 or 5 choledochojejunostomy is effective, with a near 1-year mean patency rate, but the surgery is taxing on the seriously ill.[47] Nonsurgical palliative treatment efficacy depends on the location of the obstruction, the decompression technique, the extent of decompression, and the biliary prosthesis.

Total biliary decompression is associated with longer survival[48]; thus, the treatment of lower bile duct (Bismuth I and II) lesions tend to be more successful than the treatment of Bismuth III and IV lesions because, by definition, Bismuth III and IV lesions involve the main biliary bifurcation and beyond. When compared with Bismuth I/II lesions, drainage was less successful in Bismuth III/IV lesions with less jaundice resolution (73% vs 96%), and lower mean biliary prosthesis patency (41 days vs 87 days).[49]

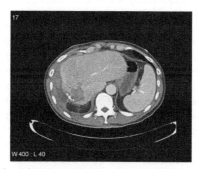

Fig. 5. Contrast-enhanced axial CT immediately after the RFA procedure described in **Fig. 4**.

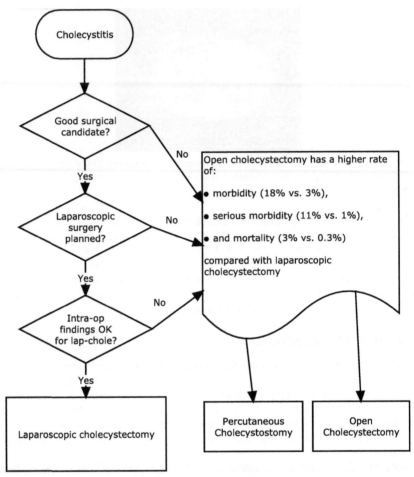

Fig. 6. Decision tree for the management of cholecystitis in frail and/or high-risk patients. See text for full discussion. Lap-chole, laparoscopic cholecystectomy.

Percutaneous or endoscopically placed self-expanding metal stents tend to have better patency rates than percutaneous or endoscopically placed plastic (usually polyethylene) drains.[50–54] The patency rate of self-expanding metal stents (30F or 10 mm in diameter) is approximately 4 months whereas the patency rate of plastic drains (10F) is only 3 months.[55] The improved patency rate of the self-expanding metal stent is likely related to the nearly 3-fold larger internal diameter of the self-expanding metal stent when compared with a plastic biliary drain, because bile tends to sludge and obstruct smaller plastic biliary drainage prostheses.[56]

According to a Cochrane Database review, self-expanding metal stents are preferred to plastic drains, although no prospective randomized trials comparing self-expanding metal stents to percutaneous plastic drains have been performed.[55] Furthermore, endoscopic self-expanding metal stent placement procedures are preferred to percutaneous stent placement procedures because percutaneous procedures are thought to have more pain and bleeding complications,[55] but this has never been verified in a randomized controlled trial. In the author's experience, the pain of the self-expanding metal stent procedure is more associated with the

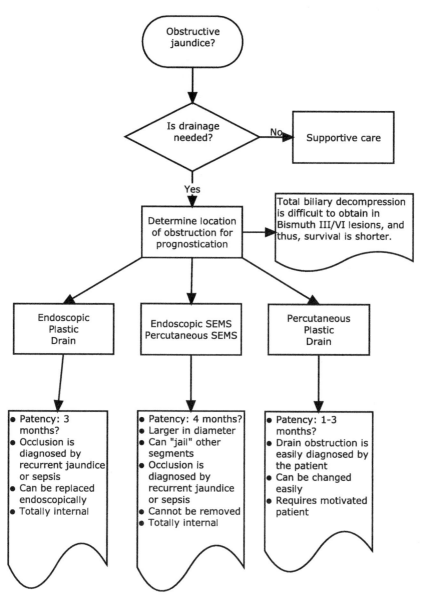

Fig. 7. Palliative biliary decompression treatment option decision tree for patients with obstructive jaundice caused by unresectable malignancies. SEMS, self-expanding metal stent.

dilitation of the self-expanding metal stent, which is required in both placement techniques. Additionally, self-expanding metal stent deployment has a tendency to jail other bile ducts, and endoscopically placed metal stents may be more problematic than percutaneously placed stents.[48] Once deployed in the biliary system, self-expanding metal stents are not removable.

Although plastic biliary drains have a higher rate of obstruction, percutaneous plastic biliary drains have 2 important advantages over endoscopically placed drains

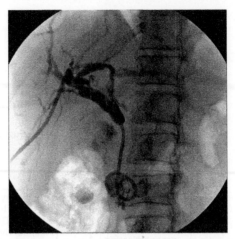

Fig. 8. Fluoroscopic cholangiography image of a percutaneous transhepatic biliary internal/external drain that decompresses the low common bile duct (Bismuth I/II) obstruction caused by metastatic pancreatic cancer. This plastic drain (10F) effectively drains all of the liver into the duodenum. Because the patient is tolerating chemotherapy well and may survive longer than 4 months, the patient has opted to keep the percutaneous drain, which can be changed easily with fluoroscopy.

(self-expanding metal stents or plastic drains) and percutaneously placed self-expanding metal stents. First, patients are aware the moment the percutaneous plastic drains become occluded because bile leaks through the end cap or around the drainage catheter. Second, these percutaneous drains can be changed easily, without general anesthesia, using basic fluoroscopy. Their basic flaw is that part of the drain is external although not necessarily attached to a drainage bag. The pain and bleeding rates associated with percutaneous plastic biliary drain placement are

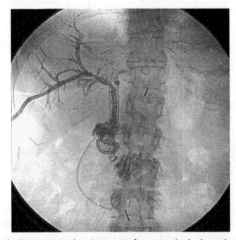

Fig. 9. Fluoroscopic cholangiography image of an occluded endoscopically placed self-expanding metal stent. Because the self-expanding metal stents are not removable, a percutaneous transhepatic biliary internal/external drain was placed through the interstices of the stent to treat the patient's recurrent biliary obstruction. Note that the right hepatic duct is jailed by the stent.

highly operator and location dependent. If the percutaneous plastic drain is placed through the subxyphoid region, the postprocedural discomfort is relatively mild. If a drain is placed through the right intercostal area, the pain is problematic for days and is accentuated by respiration. Like any other chest tube, however, the pain can be controlled with oral analgesics.

Although much has been written about survival after palliative biliary drainage, these data are suspect because patency and survival rates are subjectively determined.[55] It is likely that patients undergo one drainage procedure, then are sent to in-patient hospice when the jaundice returns—even if the jaundice is associated with sludge-mediated biliary drain occlusion, not disease progression. Therefore, percutaneous plastic drains, although associated with a short patency and more discomfort, may provide patients a longer survival because of the ease of diagnosing and changing occluded drains. Informed consent is difficult, but crucial. Although the author has seen patients live for more than 480 days with percutaneous biliary drains (usually changed every 2 months), i have also seen patents ask for in-patient hospice referral just because they did not like the external drain—painful or not.

One final caution: great care must be taken to differentiate malignant from benign bile duct obstruction. Erdogan and colleagues[57] found that 17% of patients who underwent resection for cholangiocarcinoma did not have pathologic evidence of malignancy. Half of those benign obstructions were associated with immunoglobulin G4-related sclerosing cholangitis, which looks much like cholangiocarcinoma. Treatment with intravenous steroids is effective—at least in the short term.[58–60]

GASTROSTOMY AND GASTROJEJUNOSTOMY TUBES

Feeding tubes (and gastroenteric decompression tubes) can be divided into those that are orally/nasally inserted and those that are placed directly through the skin (by surgical or fluoroscopic techniques) into the stomach or small bowel (**Fig. 10**). Oropharyngeal feeding tubes should not be used long term because they can worsen aspiration due to scarring of the transverse and oblique arytenoid muscles that cross the midline in the posterior aspect of the larynx (nasogastric tube syndrome). The dysfunctional arytenoid muscles cannot adduct the vocal cords; thus, the laryngeal inlet remains open during swallowing and aspiration results.[61]

Transcutaneous feeding tubes include gastrostomy, gastrojejunostomy, and jejunostomy tubes. Transcutaneous jejunostomy tubes (most, if not all, are placed surgically) are discussed later. Placement of a transcutaneous gastrostomy/gastrojejunostomy tube is performed on 0.8% of Caucasian and 1.7% of African American Medicare beneficiaries 85 years or older, with a 30-day, 1-year, and 3-year survival rates of 76%, 37%, and 19%.[62] Some investigators have used these data to suggest that percutaneous feeding tubes are not useful[63]; however, these survival statistics are similar to, if not better than, many other palliative care procedures presented in this article.

The indications for feeding tube insertion are a hotly debated topic that has euthanasia and racial overtones.[64] Feeding tubes are needed in those who have difficulty swallowing, but does that include people with advanced dementia or those with terminal cancer?[63] The results of feeding tube insertion studies are difficult to generalize because the results are influenced by the cognitive abilities of patients, the method of feeding (bolus vs continuous), and the lack of randomized controlled trials. Cowen and colleagues[65] found that the median survival of patients with abnormal videofluoroscopic swallowing studies was 181 days with a feeding tube compared with 33 days without a feeding tube. After correcting for age, serum albumin, and

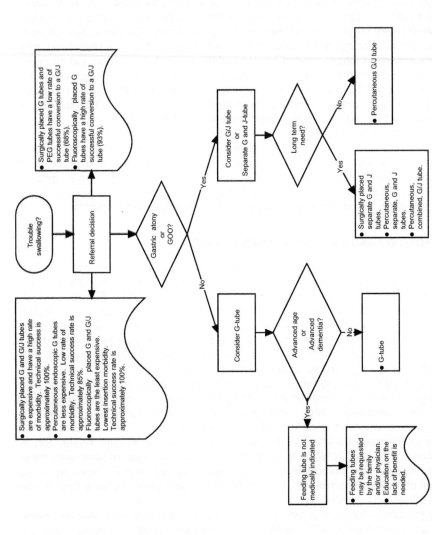

Fig. 10. Decision tree for transcutaneous feeding/decompression tubes. G, gastrostomy; G/J, gastrojejunostomy; GOO, gastric outlet obstruction; J, jejunostomy.

comorbidities, those with a percutaneous feeding tube survived twice as long. Although this seems to be recreation of the perpetual motion debate, others have shown that careful oral feeding is as effective as percutaneous feeding.[66] Nevertheless, feeding tubes cannot be expected to prevent aspiration of oral/nasal secretions, and unless the gastric part of the gastrojejunostomy tube is attached to continuous low-intermittent suction, a gastrojejunostomy does not prevent gastric reflux. Thus, feeding tubes do not prevent aspiration pneumonia in all patients, but it is likely that nutrition is better maintained.

Although no prospective randomized trials comparing fluoroscopic, endoscopic, and surgical insertion have been published, accumulated studies on the topic indicate that fluoroscopic insertion is superior to the other two types. Fluoroscopic and surgical insertions have near 100% success rates compared with endoscopic insertion (85% chance of technical success).[67,68] Considering the additional costs associated with endoscopic insertion failures, the cost of gastrostomy or gastrojejunostomy tube insertion is least expensive with the fluoroscopic technique whereas the surgical technique is the most expensive.[67] Additionally, periprocedural complication rates are least with the fluoroscopic technique (0.3%) and highest with the surgical technique (20%).[69–71] Finally, conversion of the gastrostomy tube to a gastrojejunostomy tube is more successful when the original procedure was fluoroscopic (93% chance of success) compared with the endoscopic or surgical (68% chance of success).[72]

Unless a surgically placed jejunostomy tube is needed for less than 2 weeks, the Witzel-type jejunostomy tube should be considered a technique of historical significance only. This is purely a patient care issue; many of the current jejunostomy tubes are held in place with a retention balloon, and no matter how small the retention balloon is, it tends to cause a partial bowel obstruction. Thus, a surgically created, modified chimney procedure is likely more effective for long-term enteral feeding. The short blind loop should be made just long enough to hold a retention balloon. The real advantage of this technique is that the tube can be replaced by a patient, family, or nursing staff without radiologic guidance.

PAIN MANAGEMENT

Painful bony metastases are common in patients with breast, prostate, renal, thyroid, and lung cancer. In patients who have failed bisphosponates and beta-emitting, bone seeking radiopharmaceuticals, external beam radiation is the gold standard for painful osseous lesions,[73–77] with more than 40% of patients having at least a 50% reduction of bone pain (**Fig. 11**).[73] More than half of these patients, however, have recurrent pain within a median of 15 weeks.[74] Repeat external beam radiotherapy usually cannot be performed because of local tissue toxicity. In these cases, percutaneous thermal ablation, cementoplasty with or without thermal ablation, and/or transcatheter arterial embolotherapy can be used to provide local pain control. Percutaneous thermal ablation techniques include radiofrequency ablation, cryoablation, microwave ablation, percutaneous ethanol injection, and (experimentally) laser and extracorporeal-focused high-frequency ultrasound.[78–81] RFA has been shown to effectively treat osseous pain from osteolytic or mixed osteoblastic/osteolytic metastases.[78]

Cementoplasty (or vertebroplasty when applied to a vertebral body) is a procedure where polymethylmethacrylate cement in injected under image guidance into a vertebral body compression fracture with or without prior thermal ablation.[82,83] The polymethylmethacrylate cement is cytotoxic and thermally toxic to the bone tumor and the need for prior ablative therapy is unknown. Theoretically, polymethylmethacrylate

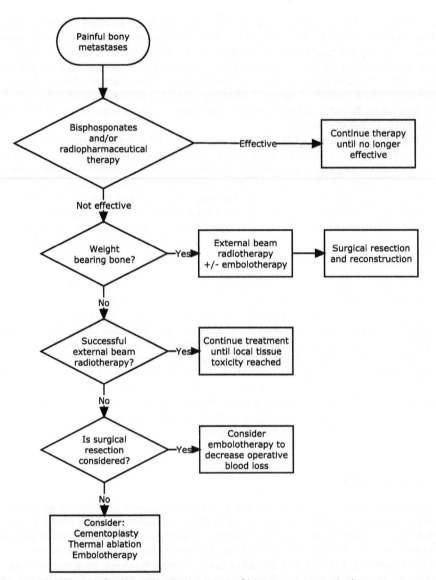

Fig. 11. Decision tree for the pain management of bony metastases. Oral, transcutaneous, and/or intravenous pain and anti-inflammatory medications are to be given concurrently with all of these procedures.

cement stabilizes the bone by cementing the microfractures, resulting in decreased pain.[78,82,83]

Surgical fixation before external beam radiotherapy is indicated for large lesions and for lesions that involve a weight-bearing bone. Depending on lesion size, location, and surgeon preference, an interventional radiologist may be asked to perform transcatheter arterial embolotherapy to limit the bleeding during the surgical extirpation and fixation.[84,85] Additionally, transarterial embolotherapy can reduce the size of viable tumor before radiation or chemotherapy and it reduces the pain associated with unresectable bone tumors.[84]

Patients with visceral pain from unresectable abdominal malignancies that are unresponsive to oral drug therapy can be offered either sympathetic neurolytic procedures[86,87] or spinal/epidural anesthetic procedures. Although percutaneous sympathetic neurolytic procedures have not been compared with spinal/epidural procedures in randomized controlled trials, neurolytic procedures may be preferable because they avoid the transcutaneous catheters and external pumps.[88] Percutaneous neurolytic procedures were found to be superior to oral/intravenous narcotics in a randomized double-blind trial by decreasing narcotic dosages and narcotic-related adverse drug effects.[89]

Celiac plexus, superior hypogastric plexus, and ganglion impar blocks are effective against midabdominal, descending colon, and rectal/perineal pain, respectively. The celiac plexus, located around the celiac artery origin, is the largest visceral plexus, containing from 1 to 5 ganglions measuring between 1.5 and 4.5 cm in diameter.[86] Absolute ethanol or 5% to 10% phenol can be injected by CT fluoroscopy and/or 2-D B-mode ultrasound via the posterior, transintervertebral disc, transabdominal aorta, and/or anterior approaches.[86,87]

TREATMENT OF REFRACTORY ASCITES

Regardless of the etiology, once a large amount of malignant ascites develops, paracentesis is effective at alleviating the pain, dyspnea, anorexia, nausea, reduced mobility, and body image dysphoria (**Fig. 12**).[90] The relief is temporary, however, with often rapid reaccumulation of the ascitic fluid.[91,92] Eventually, repeated paracenteses result in significant morbidity (bleeding, intra-abdominal organ injury, and/or infection), dehydration, malnutrition, and patient dissatisfaction. Unless orthotopic liver transplantation (OLT) is an option, all treatments for recurrent ascites are palliative.

BENIGN ASCITES

The most important diagnostic question in the treatment of ascites is the etiology: malignant or benign. Normally, ascitic fluid is produced continuously from the peritoneal serosa and absorbed by open-ended lymphatic channels in the diaphragm and is then pushed up the thoracic duct by the relatively negative pressure of the thorax.[93,94] But an increase in the resistance to lymphatic drainage by a central liver tumor (central ascites) or portal hypertension results in the production of a transudative ascites. A serum-ascites albumin gradient (SAAG) greater than 1.1 g/dL indicates ascites due to increased portal pressures with an accuracy of 97%. Unfortunately, not all diseases with benign ascites have an SAAG greater than 1.1 g/dL; peritonitis, nephrotic syndrome, and malnutrition commonly have an SAAG less than 1.1 g/dL.[94–97]

Benign ascites is responsible for 90% of the ascites cases, and refractory ascites secondary to end-stage liver disease is associated with a 20% to 50% 1-year mortality.[93] In patients with portal hypertension–associated medically refractory ascites, transjugular intrahepatic portasystemic shunting (TIPS) results in significantly better survival than repeated paracentesis.[98–100] In a study by Salerno and colleagues,[100] the 1- and 2-year survival rates for patients treated with TIPS were 77% and 59%, respectively, whereas the survival rates for those treated with repeated paracentesis were 52% and 29%, respectively. A recent meta-analysis also concluded that TIPS significantly improves transplant-free survival of cirrhosis patients with refractory ascites.[101]

Absolute contraindications to TIPS include severe right heart failure and/or pulmonary hypertension. Relative contraindications include Child-Pugh class C cirrhosis,

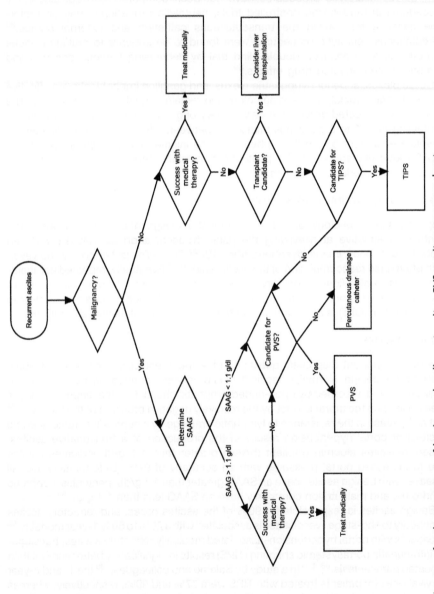

Fig. 12. Decision tree for the treatment of benign and malignant ascites. PVS, peritoneovenous shunt.

model of end-stage liver disease (MELD) score more than 22, and serum bilirubin level greater than 3 mg/dL. Other relative contra-indications include hepatic encephalopathy, polycystic liver disease, active sepsis, and chronic portal vein thrombosis.[102] Multivariate analyses demonstrate that Child-Pugh class C, MELD score greater than 25, and portosystemic pressure gradient less than 8 mm Hg after TIPS creation are the most significant predictors of mortality.[100,103]

In patients who are not candidates for TIPS, placement of a subcutaneous peritoneovenous shunt may be a good alternative to repeated paracentesis or long-term tunneled catheters.[104] Peritoneovenous shunting has been evaluated by many investigators, but to the author's knowledge no randomized trials comparing them to TIPS or tunneled drainage catheters have been completed. One study found that median survival after peritoneovenous shunting for cirrhosis was 140 days.[105] The Denver and LeVeen shunts most likely have equivalent patency rates.[104] For patients with benign ascites, contraindications to peritoneovenous shunting are thick ascites with protein levels greater than 4.5 g/L, elevated bilirubin levels, loculated ascites, coagulation disorders, congestive heart failure, and renal failure.[104]

PATHOPHYSIOLOGY AND TREATMENT OF CENTRAL ASCITES

Malignant ascites due to the central venous obstruction produces a thin transudative fluid with an SAAG greater than 1.1 g/dL. In theory, the pathophysiology of central ascites is the same as that seen in cirrhosis.[94–96] In this type of malignant ascites, diuretics and β-blockers should be effective, although the efficacy is unpredictable.[96,97] Thus, identifying this type of malignant ascites may prevent unnecessary abdominal drainage procedures. If medical treatment fails, peritoneovenous shunting or percutaneous drainage catheters are an option. Because a central hepatic tumor is the etiology of central ascites, TIPS is not an option.

TREATMENT OF CHYLOUS AND PERIPHERAL ASCITES

Malignant ascites is the abnormal accumulation of fluid in the peritoneal cavity as a consequence of cancer and is a common presentation in up to half of all patients with malignancy,[106] but it accounts for only 10% of all cases of ascites.[107] Malignant ascites is commonly associated with neoplasms of the breast, ovary, stomach, pancreas, and colon, but up to 20% are associated with an unknown primary.[108] With the exception of breast and ovarian cancer, patients with malignant ascites have a short life expectancy of 1 to 4 months.[109] Chylous ascites is caused by obstruction of the lymphatic system at or above the cisterna chyli, whereas peripheral ascites is due to peritoneal seeding.[110] Excessive protein loss due to increased microvascular permeability allows proteins and fluid to move into the peritoneum; thus, the SAAG of the ascitic fluid is low (<1.1 g/dL).[111–113]

Nontunneled percutaneous catheters are effective in single setting drainage procedures, but if left long-term, they are prone to infection, accidental removal, leakage, and occlusion. Long-term drainage can be obtained from tunneled drainage catheters: the PleurX catheter (CareFusion, San Diego, CA, USA) and the Aspira catheter (Bard Access Systems, Salt Lake City, UT, USA). Both use a Dacron cuff in the subcutaneous fat to decrease the chance of infection, and both have a special valve that prevents leakage and/or bacterial contamination.

Peritoneovenous shunting is likely to be superior to repeated paracentesis if a patient's survival is more than 1 to 2 months. After peritoneovenous shunting, abdominal girth and red blood cell concentration decrease significantly, whereas performance score, possible discharge rate, and median survival increase significantly compared with repeated paracenteses.[92] Likely due to the short life expectancy of patients with malignant ascites treated with peritoneovenous shunting, necropsy studies have not found hematologically disseminated metastases.[92,104–115]

In a prospective study of 34 patients with malignant ascites who were treated with a tunnelled drainage catheter, 85% required no catheter interventions before removal/death, whereas bloating and abdominal discomfort were significantly reduced at 2 and 8 weeks.[116]

RECURRENT PLEURAL EFFUSIONS

After tube thoracostomy or thoracentesis, the finding of incomplete lung expansion is suggestive of either a trapped lung (pneumothorax ex vacuo) or pneumothorax.[117] This intrathoracic space invariably raises alarms from diagnostic radiologists, but a clinician can differentiate a pneumothorax ex vacuo from a pneumothorax based on the results of the thoracentesis; if no air was aspirated from the pleural space during the thoracentesis, the chest radiograph most likely depicts a pneumothorax ex vacuo not a pneumothorax. Placing a tube thoracostomy does not re-expand a trapped lung—no matter how much suction is applied. Furthermore, fluid returns to fill this space for a long as the pleural space exists.[117,118] If the pleural fluid was sterile before placing a long-term nontunneled chest tube, the pleural space eventually becomes contaminated and leads to empyema development.

TREATMENT OF RECURRENT, SYMPTOMATIC, STERILE PLEURAL EFFUSION IN FRAIL PATIENTS

If a trapped lung (chronic empyema thoracis) is discovered after thoracentesis, and fibrinolytic therapy fails to re-expand the lung, then a long-term chest tube or open window thoracotomy is acceptable treatment (**Fig. 13**).[118] In this case, the lung is fixed and pleural suction is not necessary. Standard surgical therapy, decortication, muscle/omental flap transposition (plombage), and thoracoplasty are all too morbid

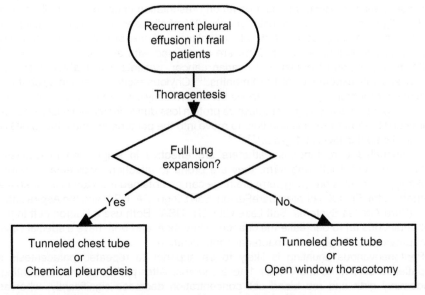

Fig. 13. Decision tree for the treatment of benign pleural effusions.

for frail patients. In cases of chronic empyema thoracis, bismuth paste plombage may be an effective treatment,[119] but this does not treat the patient's dyspnea. Alternatively, if the lung expands fully after thoracentesis, clinicians have the option of a long-term tunneled chest drain or chemical pleurodesis to prevent recurrence of the pleural effusion.

TREATMENT OF RECURRENT, STERILE, MALIGNANT PLEURAL EFFUSIONS

Again, thoracentesis or tube thoracostomy is needed to determine if the lung is trapped beneath a layer of fibrin or malignant cells. If a trapped lung is diagnosed, then long-term tube thoracostomy is the only real option (**Figs. 14–16**).[117] Open window thoracostomy is a suboptimal treatment, because eventually the tumor grows out through the chest wall defect, making dressing changes unpleasant. Because of the short life expectancy, decortication, muscle/omental plombage, and thoracoplasty are inappropriate.

If, however, the lung fully expands, then the clinician can use either a tunneled chest drain or chemical pleurodesis. Currently there are 2 Food and Drug Administration (FDA)-approved tunneled chest catheters for long-term drainage of malignant pleural effusions: the PleurX catheter and the Aspira catheter. Both have a special valve at the end of the external part of the drainage catheter that prevents leakage of air and fluid. Studies have shown that the tunneled pleural cathers are effective, with pleurodesis occurring in at least 42%.[120] Although both catheters are easy to insert, our interventional radiology group prefers the Aspira system because the insertion kit comes with 20 drainage bags; the PleurX kit does not come with extra vacuum bottles—patients must order them.

As long as the lung is fully expanded, chemical pleurodesis obliterates the pleural space and prevents recurrence of the pleural effusion.[121] Although bleomycin and doxycycline have been used with moderate success for chemical pleurodesis, they are associated with significant patient discomfort. Administration of a talc slurry (4 g talc, 50 mL 1% lidocaine, and 50 mL saline), placed through a large chest tube (28F or larger) is effective and well tolerated. Minimal patient discomfort and a mild fever are the only side effects commonly seen. Once pleural drainage has dropped below 100 mL per day (which usually takes 3 to 7 days), the chest tube can be removed. Using this protocol, recurrence of the pleural effusion is rare (<10%).[121–123] The medical grade talc available today is sorted to remove the smallest particles; however, this was not always the case.[124] Studies have shown that these small particles were responsible for clinically apparent hypoxia,[125] respiratory distress–like syndromes,[126] and death (2%).[127,128]

A comparison of talc pleurodesis and long-term tunneled chest catheter in the treatment of malignant pleural effusion found that the cost and effectiveness were nearly equal.[129] But, because talc pleurodesis requires a prolonged hospital stay, long-term tunneled chest catheter placement was more cost effective (and patient friendly) when life expectancy was 6 weeks or less. Furthermore, Ozyurtkan and colleagues[123] found that malignant pleural effusions associated with certain malignancies are associated with early mortality (lung, stomach, soft tissue, bladder, esophagus, prostate, cervix, and lymphoma); thus, a long-term tunneled chest catheter may be more appropriate in these cases.

PALLIATIVE THERAPY FOR HEPATOCELLULAR CARCINOMA
Early HCC

HCC is an increasingly common disease[130] and without treatment, life expectancy is short,[131] but in contrast to other types of malignancy, patients with HCC die of liver

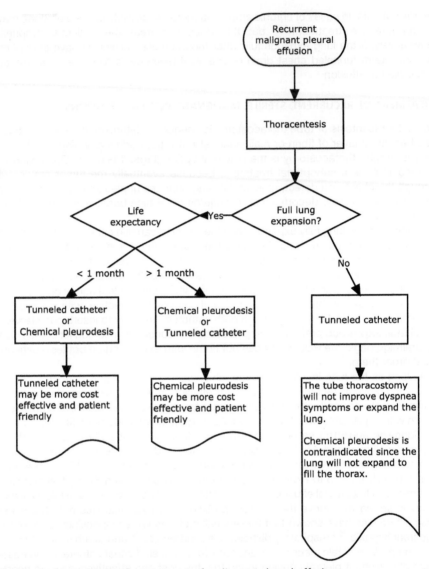

Fig. 14. Decision tree for the treatment of malignant pleural effusions.

failure (due to progressive cirrhosis or tumor burden) not disseminated disease (**Fig. 17**). Patients with early HCC are those that meet the Milan criteria for OLT (3 tumors <3 cm or 1 <5 cm).[132] Without liver transplantation, recurrence is common whether the locoregional treatment is surgery or ablative therapy.[131]

Resection may no longer be the only effective locoregional therapy for HCC.[133] Thermal ablation (using radiofrequency or microwave energy) has been shown in 2 prospective randomized controlled trials to provide equivalent intermediate-term overall survival to resective therapy in patients with small HCC tumors.[134,135] A study by Chen and colleagues[134] used the Milan criteria, whereas a study by Lü and colleagues[135] restricted patients to a single tumor less than 5 cm. These studies found thermal ablation and surgical resection 1-, 2-, 3- and 4-year survival rates of

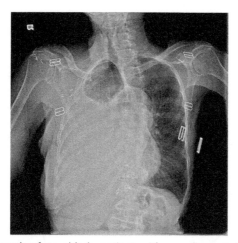

Fig. 15. Chest radiograph of an elderly patient with a malignant right pleural effusion admitted with fever and chills.

approximately 95%, 84%, 79%, and 68% versus 92%, 84%, 79%, and 64%, respectively (the study by Lü gave survival data to only 3 years). Three additional retrospective cohort studies on cirrhotic patients with small HCC lesions[136–138] and at least one report involving OLT patients with HCC recurrence[139] yielded similar results.

Despite the fact that HCC is a multifocal disease with a high recurrence rate, palliative therapy with ethanol or thermal ablation is indicated over supportive care.[131] Survival depends on the amount of residual functioning liver (Child-Pugh class is more predictive than the Okuda staging) and the size and number of HCC tumors.

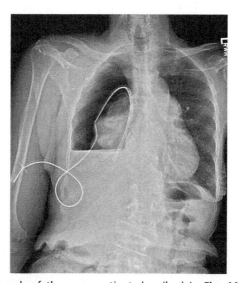

Fig. 16. Chest radiograph of the same patient described in **Fig. 14** after placement of a tunneled chest drain. Because the lung is trapped under a layer of malignant/fibrous tissue, the lung will not be able to re-expand and the patient's dyspnea will not resolve. The chest radiograph depicts a pneumothorax ex vacuo, not a pneumothorax. No amount of suction will expand this lung.

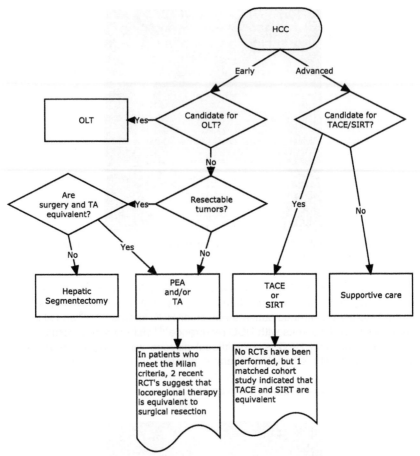

Fig. 17. Decision tree for the treatment of early and advanced HCC. PEA, percutaneous ethanol ablation; RCT, randomized controlled trial; TA, thermal ablation.

For patients who fulfill the Milan criteria for OLT, the 2-year survival rates for those who only receive supportive care are 33%, 17%, and 0% for Child-Pugh classes A, B, and C, respectively. The 2-year survival rates for those receiving locoregional therapy, however, are 65%, 51%, and 15%, respectively. This difference was statistically significant for all Child-Pugh classes.

Percutaneous ethanol, injected with ultrasound, CT, or MRI guidance, is also an effective therapy in HCC because the HCC tumors are relatively soft compared with the hard cirrhotic surrounding liver. In 2003, Lencioni and colleagues[140] published a prospective randomized trial comparing RFA and percutaneous ethanol ablation as locoregional therapy for small HCC tumors in cirrhotic patients. For the RFA group, the 1- and 2-year overall survival rates were 100% and 98%, whereas the 1- and 2-year survival rates for the percutaneous ethanol ablation group were 96% and 88% (relative risk 0.20; 95% CI, 0.02–1.69; $P = .138$). The 1- and 2-year event-free survival rates were 86% and 46% in the RFA group versus 77% and 43% for the percutaneous ethanol ablation group ($P = .012$). In 2008, Brunello and colleagues[141] published an intention-to-treat study comparing percutaneous ethanol ablation and RFA in patients with small HCC nodules (15 to 30 mm) with Child-Pugh class A or B cirrhosis. The

1-year complete response rate was 65.7% and 36.2% in patients treated by RFA and percutaneous ethanol ablation, respectively ($P = .0005$), but the overall survival rate was not significantly different (adjusted hazard ratio 0.88; 95% CI, 0.50–1.53).

Percutaneous ethanol ablation and RFA may need to be used together, because RFA efficacy is limited by the heat sink of large vascular structures. In 2007, Zhang and colleagues[142] published a prospective randomized trial comparing RFA to RFA plus percutaneous ethanol ablation. Survival rates in the RFA plus percutaneous ethanol ablation group at 1, 2, 3, 4, and 5 years were 95.4%, 89.2%, 75.8%, 63.3%, and 49.3% compared with RFA alone group, which had survival rates of 89.6%, 68.7%, 58.4%, 50.3%, and 35.9%. The RFA plus percutaneous ethanol ablation treatment was better in the 3.1- to 5.0-cm tumor group ($P = .03$) but not for other tumor sizes ($\leq$3.0 cm; $P = .44$ and 5.1–7.0 cm; $P = .70$). Based on this study, Zhang and colleagues concluded that RFA plus percutaneous ethanol ablation resulted in better local tumor control and long-term survival compared with RFA alone. Treatment type and tumor size were significant prognostic factors for local recurrence.

The compounded annual growth rate of percutaneous ablative procedures for liver tumors was 12% from 2002 to 2008.[143] This growth rate has raised some concerns about US patients with potentially curable HCC treated with palliative locoregional therapy[144]; data show that the number of patients undergoing resection is unchanged (8.5% to 9.2%), whereas the number of patients treated with locoregional therapy increased (3.2% to 12.1%) between 1998 and 2005. The position of the Society of Interventional Radiology is that "percutaneous RF ablation of hepatic tumors is a safe and effective treatment for selected patients with HCC ...."[145]

Advanced HCC

TACE, described in detail previously,[146–149] has been performed for more than 30 years and is the most acceptable form of treatment for advanced HCC. Previous randomized controlled trials comparing TACE to supportive care have failed to show any survival benefit to TACE over supportive care, but this may have been due to the high rate of TACE-induced liver failure in some of these studies. There is, however, now level 1 support for TACE for the treatment of unresectable HCC.[16,150] In a study by Llovet, and colleagues,[16] survival rates at 1 and 2 years were 82% and 63% for TACE, yet 63% and 27% for the supportive care control group ($P = .009$). Treatment allocation was the only variable independently associated with survival ($P = .02$). In a study by Lo and colleagues,[150] patients treated with TACE had a significantly better survival than patients treated with supportive care. The 1-, 2-, and 3-year overall survival rates for patients treated with TACE were 57%, 31%, and 26% compared with 32%, 11%, and 3% for those treated with supportive care, respectively ($P = .002$). Even when prognostic variables, determined by univariate analysis, were controlled for, TACE was significantly better than supportive care (relative risk 0.49; 95% CI, 0.29–0.81; $P = .006$). The Society of Interventional Radiology position statement on TACE for hepatic tumors is that "[It] is a safe, proven, and effective technique for the treatment of a number of malignancies, including HCC..."[146]

Because patients with HCC generally die of liver failure rather than widespread metastatic disease,[151] current therapy limits TACE to patients with Child-Pugh class A and B cirrhosis with a serum of 3.4 g/dL or greater[149] and a serum total bilirubin of less than 3 mg/dL.[152] Furthermore, patients do not tolerate TACE if more than 50% of the liver is replaced with tumor, the serum total bilirubin is greater than 2 mg/dL, the lactate dehydrogenase is greater than 425 mg/dL, and the aspartate aminotransferase is more than 100 IU/L (all 4 must be present).[149,153]

SELECTIVE INTERNAL RADIOTHERAPY

An alternative form of therapy for advanced HCC, not proved by randomized controlled trials, is SIRT. TheraSphere particles (MDS Nordion, Kanata, Ontario, Canada), were approved by the US FDA for the treatment in unresectable HCC in 1999 under the provisions of humanitarian device exemption H9800006.[154] TheraSpheres are glass microspheres 20 to 30 μm in size with yttrium 90. One 3-GBq vial contains 1.2 million particles, with 2500 Bq of radioactivity per microsphere (TheraSphere package insert). The arterial embolic effect is minimal; thus, tumor ischemia is not a major part of this treatment. Relative contraindications to SIRT include limited hepatic reserve, compromised portal vein, and prior radiation therapy to the liver.[25]

A recent phase II trial of SIRT treatment of HCC found that regardless of the amount of tumor burden, the tumor response to yttrium 90 was similar.[151] When patients were divided into low, medium, and high radioembolization risk groups, median survival rates were 46.5 months, 16.9 months, and 11.1 months, respectively. Median survival rates by Okuda stage were 24.4 months and 12.5 months for stages I and II, and median survival by Child-Pugh class was 22.7 months for class A and 13.6 months for class B/C. Another trial found 5 liver reserve variables that can be used to stratify patients into low- and high-risk groups.[155] Any of the following liver reserve risk variables places a patient into the high-risk group for 3-month mortality after SIRT: infiltrative disease, bulky disease (tumor burden is ≥70% of the liver), AST and ALT greater than 5 times upper limit of normal, tumor burden greater than or equal to 50%, and albumin less than 3 g/dL, and bilirubin greater than or equal to 2 mg/dL. Three-month survival rate was 51% in the high-risk group and 93% in the low-risk group.

Although there are no randomized controlled trials to support the use of SIRT, a consensus panel report from the Radioembolization Brachytherapy Oncology Consortium "believes that there is sufficient evidence to support the safety and effectiveness of yttrium 90 microsphere therapy in selected patients [with primary or secondary hepatic tumors]."[154]

COLORECTAL LIVER METASTASES

Up to 60% of patients with colorectal cancer develop hepatic metastases at some point in their lives (**Fig. 18**).[156] CRLM patients who are untreated have a median survival of approximately 5 months and no chance of living 5 years.[157] Although fewer than 30% of patients have resectable disease,[158] surgery is the only accepted curative treatment for colorectal liver metastases.[159] If completely resected, the mean 5-year survival for patients with 3 or fewer CRLM is 39%, whereas the mean 5-year survival for patients with 4 or more CRLM is 17.1%.[159] Partial hepatectomy is a relatively morbid surgical procedure; the overall mortality for hepatic resection is 5.8%, but the in-hospital mortality rate for 70- to 80-year-old patients undergoing hepatic resection for CRLM is 8.9%.[160] Assuming no new metachronous lesions are found, hepatic metastasectomy is a cost-effective option for selected patients with metachronous colorectal carcinoma metastases limited to the liver at $32,000 per quality-adjusted life year, including follow-up.[161] Neoadjuvant chemotherapy is currently offered to patients with resectable CRLM, and chemotherapy is used to downsize CRLM to increase the percentage of patients who are resectable.[162] Multiple chemotherapy protocol options are now available.[163]

RFA of CRLM

Excellent reviews of locoregional therapy of CRLM with RFA have been published recently.[29,145] Although no randomized controlled trials have been published, a review

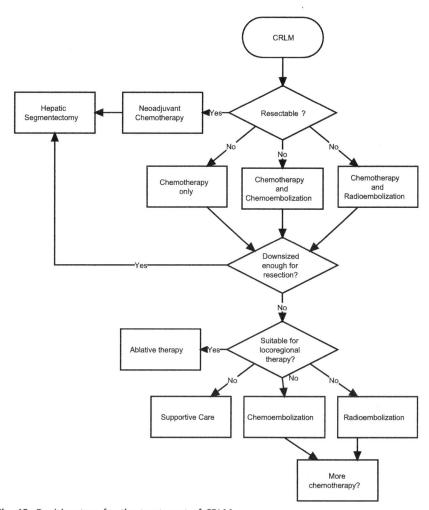

Fig. 18. Decision tree for the treatment of CRLM.

of the literature by Mulier and colleagues[164] suggests that open RFA is equivalent to resection for colorectal liver metastases less than 3 cm. Additionally, long-term control of CRLM with RFA can be achieved in 40% to 98% of tumors, with a 5-year survival rate of 14% to 55%. The treatment of CRLM with RFA has a reported mortality of 0% to 2% with a major complication rate of 6% to 9%.[165,166] The Society of Interventional Radiology 2009 position statement supports the use of RFA in selected patients with CRLM.[145]

Livraghi and colleagues[167] performed a trial that used RFA in a test-of-time approach to see if other CRLM appear in other regions. Complete necrosis was obtained in 60% of patients and 63% of lesions. Of the patients who had complete necrosis, only 30% remained disease-free and 70% developed new lesions elsewhere. No patients became unresectable due to growth of the ablated tumors, but 98% were spared surgical resection because either they did not develop metachronous tumors (and the initial RFA was definitive therapy) or they developed disease progression elsewhere.

The best outcomes after RFA involve situations with solitary CRLM lesions.[168–170] Because most thermal ablation devices cause coagulation necrosis up to 4 cm, the failure rates of RFA increase significantly if the tumors are greater than 3 cm in diameter.[169,170] RFA near large blood vessels has a high rate of failure because of the heat sink, and RFA near the hilum can cause major bile duct injury. Because RFA is an image-guided technique, the success of the procedures relates to the imaging. Because of respiratory motion, 2-D B-mode ultrasound is often the best imaging technique; thus, RFA performed during an open laparotomy has the lowest local recurrence rates.[171]

TACE for CRLM

The Society of Interventional Radiology 2009 position statement on transcatheter liver therapy states that TACE has a palliative role for patients with colon carcinoma liver metastases, although a survival of at least 12 months is needed to make this cost effective.[146] Survival is affected by performance status; for those with Eastern Cooperative Oncology Group performance status of 0 or 1, the median survival is 24 months versus 3 months with a performance status of 2. Furthermore, no extrahepatic disease at the time of TACE yielded a median survival of 14 months versus 3 months for those with extrahepatic disease.[172] Using TACE with cisplatin, doxorubicin, mitomycin, lipiodol, and polyvinyl alcohol particles, the 1-, 2-, and 3-year survival rates were 86%, 55%, and 23%, with a median survival of 24 months.[173]

SIRT for CRLM

SIR-Spheres (SirTeX Medical, Lane Cove, New South Wales, Australia) were approved by the FDA for use in CRLM in 2002 but must be given with concurrent fluorodeoxyuridine infusion.[154,174–176] SIR-Spheres are resin microspheres ranging in size from 20 to 60 μm. One 3-Gbq vial contains 40 to 80 million particles; activity per microsphere is 50 Bq (SIR-Spheres package insert). Because of the number of particles, they impart an embolic effect; thus, tumor ischemia is an important part of this treatment.[25] The pretreatment evaluation (angiography and lung shunt fraction determination) and the risks of off-target embolotherapy with yttrium 90 are the same as described for Thera-Sphere treatment of HCC.[25]

Survival after radioembolization depends on the amount of CRLM in the liver, the presence of extrahepatic disease, performance status, function of the residual liver, and carcinoembryonic antigen level changes.[28,177] In a phase III randomized trial comparing SIRT plus hepatic arterial chemotherapy with floxuridine versus the same hepatic artery chemotherapy, no statistically significant survival differences were noted, but there was a significant increase in tumor volume responses (50% vs 24%; $P = .03$) and progression-free survival (16 months vs 10 months; $P = .001$).[178] In a phase II randomized trial of systemic chemotherapy (fluorouracil and leucovorin) with or without a singe SIRT treatment, the addition of a single SIRT treatment increased treatment response ($P<.001$), time to disease progression (19 months vs 4 months; $P<.0005$), and median survival (29 months vs 13 months; $P = .02$).[179]

SUMMARY

Image-guided palliative procedures, such as those discussed in this article, are performed by surgeons and/or interventional radiologists. These procedures, which are percutaneous by nature, are designed to prolong life and minimize pain and suffering with the smallest physiologic challenge. Unfortunately, few of these procedures have been validated by randomized controlled trials and none has been comparatively evaluated to other palliative care options, so their integration into end-of-life care is still in question. As the baby boom generation ages, the number of people needing these types of microinvasive procedures will increase dramatically, and determining the cost and effectiveness of these palliative care procedures will become a national priority.

REFERENCES

1. McCullough HK, Bain RM, Clark HP, et al. The interventional radiologist as a palliative care sub-specialist: providing symptom relief when cure is not possible. AJR 2010;196:462–7.
2. Baerlocher MO, Asch MR. Interventional radiology in palliative care. CMAJ 2007;176(6):762–3.
3. Shem S. The house of god. New York: Dell Publishing Co, Inc; 1978.
4. Barnato AE, Herndon MB, Anthony DL, et al. Are regional variations in end-of-life care intensity explained by patient preferences? Med Care 2007;45:386–93.
5. Fried TR, Byers AL, Gallo WT, et al. Prospective study of health status preferences and changes over time in older adults. Arch Intern Med 2006;166: 890–5.
6. Whiteneck GG, Carter RE, Charlifue SW, et al. A collaborative study of high quadriplegia. Denver (CO): National Institute of Handicapped Research; 1985.
7. Finucane TE. How gravely ill becomes dying: a key to end-of-life care. JAMA 1999;282:1670–2.
8. Institute of medicine 100 initial priority topics for comparative effectiveness research. Available at: http://www.iom.edu/CMS. Accessed August 15, 2010.
9. Earle CC, Chapman RH, Baker CS, et al. Systematic overview of cost-utility assessments in oncology. J Clin Oncol 2000;18:3302–17.
10. Weinstein MC, Skinner JA. Comparative effectiveness and health care spending—implications for reform. N Engl J Med 2010;362:460–5.
11. Sutherland JM, Fisher ES, Skinner JS. Getting past denial—the high cost of health care in the United States. N Engl J Med 2009;361:1227–30.
12. Kheterpal S. Perioperative comparative effectiveness research. An opportunity calling. Anesthesiology 2009;111:1180–2.
13. Pandharipande PV, Gazelle GS. Comparative effectiveness research: what it means for radiology. Radiology 2009;253:600–5.
14. Hattery RR, Leibel SA, Lewis FR, et al. Memorandum of understanding between ABS and ABR concerning the ABS application for primary certification in vascular surgery. 2004. Available at: http://www.members.SIRweb.org./members/resources. cfm. Accessed August 21, 2010.
15. Lien WM, Ackerman NB. The blood supply of experimental liver metastases II: a microcirculatory study of the normal and tumor vessels of the liver with the use of perfused silicone rubber. Surgery 1970;68:334–40.
16. Llovet JM, Real MI, Montaña X, et al. Arterial embolization or chemoembolization versus symptomatic treatment in patients with unresectable hepatocellular carcinoma: a randomized controlled trial. Lancet 2002;359:1734–9.
17. Kono T. Targeting cancer chemotherapeutic agents by use of lipiodol contrast medium. Cancer 1990;66:1897–903.
18. Egawa H, Maki A, Mori K, et al. Effects of intra-arterial chemotherapy with a new lipophilic anticancer agent, estradiol-chlorambucil (KM2210), dissolved in lipiodol on experimental liver tumor in rats. J Surg Oncol 1990;44:109–14.

19. Groupe De'Etude Et De Traitement Du carcinoma Hepatocellulaire. A comparison of lipiodol chemoembolization and conservative treatment for unresectable hepatocellular carcinoma. N Engl J Med 1995;332:1256–61.
20. Bronowicki JP, Vetter D, Dumas F, et al. Transcatheter oily chemoembolization for hepatocellular carcinoma. A 4-year study of 127 French patients. Cancer 1994;74:16–24.
21. Nakakuma K, Tashiro S, Hiraoka T, et al. Studies on anticancer treatment with an oily anticancer drug injected into the ligated feeding hepatic artery for liver cancer. Cancer 1983;52:2193–200.
22. Kim P, Prapong W, Sze DY, et al. Treatment of hepatocellular carcinoma with sub-selective transcatheter arterial oily chemoinfusion. Tech Vasc Interv Radiol 2002;5:127–31.
23. Lau WY, Leung WT, Ho LS, et al. Treatment of inoperable hepatocellular carcinoma with intrahepatic arterial yttrium-90 microspheres: a phase I and II study. Br J Cancer 1994;70:994–9.
24. Phillips R, Karnofsky DA, Hamilton LD, et al. Roentgen therapy of hepatic metastases. Am J Roentgenol Radium Ther Nucl Med 1954;71:826–34.
25. Riaz A, Lewandowski RJ, Kulik LM, et al. Complications following radioembolization with yttrium-90 microspheres: a comprehensive literature review. J Vasc Interv Radiol 2009;20:1121–30.
26. Lau WY, Ho S, Leung TW, et al. Selective internal radiation therapy for nonresectable hepatocellular carcinoma with intraarterial infusion of 90-yttrium microspheres. Int J Radiat Oncol Biol Phys 1998;40:583–92.
27. Kennedy AS, Nutting C, Coldwell D, et al. Pathologic response and microdosimetry of 90Y microspheres in man: review of four explanted whole livers. Int J Radiat Oncol Biol Phys 2004;60:1552–63.
28. Mulcahy MF, Lewandowski RJ, Ibrahim SM, et al. Radioembolization of colorectal hepatic metastases using yttrium-90 microspheres. Cancer 2009;115:1849–58.
29. Hong K, Georgiades C. Radiofrequency ablation: mechanism of action and devices. J Vasc Interv Radiol 2010;21:S179–86.
30. Lubner MG, Brace CL, Hinshaw JL, et al. Microwave tumor ablation: mechanism of action, clinical results, and devices. J Vasc Interv Radiol 2010;21:S192–203.
31. Erinjeri JP, Clark TW. Cryoablation: mechanism of action and devices. J Vasc Interv Radiol 2010;21:S187–91.
32. Korpan NN. A history of cryosurgery: its development and future. J Am Coll Surg 2007;204:314–24.
33. Clark TW. Chemical ablation of liver cancer. Tech Vasc Interv Radiol 2007;10:58–63.
34. US Department of Health and Human Services, National Center for Health Statistics. National health statistics reports: 2006 national hospital discharge survey. Washington, DC: US Department of Health and Human Services; 2008.
35. US Department of Health and Human Services, National Center for Health Statistics. National health statistics reports: ambulatory surgery in the United States, 2006. Washington, DC: US Department of Health and Human Services; 2009.
36. Murphy MM, Ng SC, Simons JP, et al. Predictors of major complications after laparoscopic cholecystectomy: surgeon, hospital, or patient? J Am Coll Surg 2010;211:73–80.
37. Ingraham AM, Cohen ME, Ko CY, et al. A current profile and assessment of North American cholecystectomy: results from the American College of Surgeons

National Surgical Quality Improvement Program. J Am Coll Surg 2010;211: 176–86.

38. Riall TS, Zhang D, Townsend CM, et al. Failure to perform cholecystectomy for acute cholecystitis in elderly patients is associated with increased morbidity, mortality, and cost. J AM Coll Surg 2010;210:668–79.
39. Rader RW. Ultrasonically guided percutaneous catheter drainage for gallbladder empyema. Diagn Imaging 1980;49:330–3.
40. Welschbillig-Meunier K, Pessaux P, Lebigot J, et al. Percutaneous cholesystostomy for high-risk patients with acute cholecystitis. Surg Endosc 2005;19: 1256–9.
41. Spira RM, Nissan A, Zamir O, et al. Percutaneous transhepatic cholecystostomy and delayed laparoscopic cholecystectomy in critically ill patients with acute calculus cholecystitis. Am J Surg 2002;183:62–6.
42. Leveau P, Anderson E, Carlgren I, et al. Percutaneous cholecystostomy: a bridge to surgery or definite management of acute cholecystitis in high-risk patients. Scand J Gastroenterol 2008;43:593–6.
43. Tseng JY, Yang MJ, Yang CC, et al. Acute cholecystitis during pregnancy: what is the best approach? Taiwan J Obstet Gynecol 2009;48:305–7.
44. Allmendinger N, Hallisey MJ, Ohki SK, et al. Percutaneous cholecystostomy treatment of acute cholecystitis in pregnancy. Obstet Gynecol 1995;86:653–4.
45. Neumayer L, Marcaccio M, Visser B, et al. Management of biliary tract disease during pregnancy. J Am Coll Surg 2010;210:367–9.
46. Requarth JA. Ultrasound guided percutaneous cholecystostomy in pregnancy. J Am Coll Surg 2010;211:145.
47. Jarnagin WR, Burke E, Powers EA, et al. Intrahepatic biliary bypass provides effective palliation in selected patients with malignant obstruction at the hepatic duct confluence. Am J Surg 1998;175:453–60.
48. Paik WH, Park YS, Hwang JH, et al. Palliative treatment with self-expandable metallic stents in patients with advanced type III or IV hilar cholangiocarcinoma: a percutaneous versus endoscopic approach. Gastrointest Endosc 2009;69: 55–62.
49. Rerknimitr R, Kladcharoen N, Mahachai V, et al. Result of endoscopic biliary drainage in hilar cholangiocarcinoma. J Clin Gastroenterol 2004;38: 518–23.
50. Shinchi H, Takao S, Nishida H, et al. Length and quality of survival following external beam radiotherapy combined with expandable metallic stent for unresectable hilar cholangiocarcinoma. J Surg Oncol 2000;75:89–94.
51. Kloek JJ, van der Gaag NA, Aziz Y, et al. Endoscopic and percutaneous preoperative biliary drainage in patients with suspected hilar cholangiocarcinoma. J Gastrointest Surg 2010;14:119–25.
52. Pinol V, Castells A, Bordas JM, et al. Percutaneous self-expanding metal stents versus endoscopic polyethylene endoprosthesis for treating malignant biliary obstruction: randomized clinical trial. Radiology 2002;225:27–34.
53. Speer AG, Cotton PB, Russel RC, et al. Randomized trial of endoscopic versus percutaneous stent insertion in malignant obstructive jaundice. Lancet 1987; 2(8550):57–62.
54. Gilbert DA, DiMarino AJ, Jensen DM, et al. Status evaluation: biliary stents. American Society for Gastrointestinal Endoscopy. Technology assessment committee. Gastrointest Endosc 1992;38:750–2.
55. Moss AC, Morris E, MacMathuna P. Palliative biliary stents for obstructing pancreatic carcinoma. Cochrane Database Syst Rev 2006;2:CD004200.

56. Coene PP, Groen AK, Cheng J, et al. Clogging of biliary endoprosthesis: a new perspective. Gut 1990;31:913–7.
57. Erdogan D, Kloek JJ, ten Kate FJ, et al. Immunoglobulin G4-related sclerosing cholangitis in patients resected for presumed malignant bile duct strictures. Br J Surg 2008;95:727–34.
58. Bjornsson E, Chari ST, Smyrk TC, et al. Immunoglobulin G4 associated cholangitis: description of an emerging clinical entity based on review of the literature. Hepatology 2007;45:1547–54.
59. Ghazale A, Chari ST, Zhang L, et al. Immunoglobulin G4-associated cholangitis: clinical profile and response to therapy. Gastroenterology 2008;134:706–15.
60. Church NI, Pereira SP, Deheragoda MG, et al. Autoimmune pancreatitis: clinical and radiological features and objective response to steroid therapy in a UK series. Am J Gastroenterol 2007;102:2417–25.
61. Moore KL. In: Clinically oriented anatomy. Baltimore (MD): Williams & Wilkins; 1980. p. 1185. Chapter 9.
62. Grant MD, Rudberg MA, Brody JA. Gastrostomy placement and mortality amoung hospitalized Medicare beneficiaries. JAMA 1998;279:1973–6.
63. Finucane TE, Christmas C, Travis K. Tube feeding in patients with advanced dementia. A review of the evidence. JAMA 1999;282:1365–70.
64. Welch LC, Teno JM, Mor V. End-of-life care in black and white: race matters for medical care of dying patients and their families. J Am Geriatr Soc 2005;53: 1145–53.
65. Cowen ME, Simpson SL, Vettese TE. Survival estimates for patients with abnormal swallowing studies. J Gen Intern Med 1997;12:88–94.
66. Franzoni S, Frisoni GB, Boffelli S, et al. Good nutritional oral intake is associated with equal survival in demented and nondemented very old patients. J Am Geriatr Soc 1996;44:1366–70.
67. Barkmeier JM, Trerotola SO, Wiebke EA, et al. Percutaneous radiologic, surgical endoscopic, and percutaneous endoscopic gastrostomy/gastrojejunostomy: comparative study and cost analysis. Cardiovasc Intervent Radiol 1998;21:324–8.
68. Blondet A, Lebigot J, Nicolas G, et al. Radiologic versus endoscopic placement of percutaneous gastrostomy in amyotrophic lateral sclerosis: multivariate analysis of tolerance, efficacy, and survival. J Vasc Interv Radiol 2010;21:527–33.
69. Wollman B, D'Agostino HB, Walus-Wigle JR, et al. Radiologic, endoscopic, and surgical gastrostomy: an institutional evaluation and meta-analysis of the literature. Radiology 1995;197:699–704.
70. Ho CS, Yee AC, McPherson R. Complications of surgical and percutaneous nonendoscopic gastrostomy: review of 233 patients. Gastroenterology 1988;95:1206–10.
71. Ho SGF, Marchinkow LO, Legiehn GM, et al. Radiologic percutaneous gastrostomy. Clin Radiol 2001;56:902–10.
72. Kim CY, Patel MB, Miller MJ, et al. Gastrostomy-to-gastrojejunostomy tube conversion: impact of the method of original gastrostomy tube placement. J Vasc Interv Radiol 2010;21:1031–7.
73. Agarawal JP, Swangsilpa T, van der Linden Y, et al. The role of external beam radiotherapy in the management of bone metastases. Clin Oncol (R Coll Radiol) 2006;18:747–60.
74. Tong D, Gillick L, Hendrickson FR. The palliation of symptomatic osseous metastases: final results of the Study by the Radiation Therapy Oncology Group. Cancer 1982;50:893–9.
75. Silberstein EB, Eugene L, Saenger SR. Painful osteoblastic metastases: the role of nuclear medicine. Oncology 2001;15:157–63.

76. Kirkbride P. The role of radiation therapy in palliative care. J Palliat Care 1995; 11:19–26.

77. Hellman RS, Krasnow AZ. Radionuclide therapy for palliation of pain due to osteoblastic metastases. J Palliat Med 1998;1:277–83.

78. Kurup AN, Callstrom MR. Ablation of skeletal metastases: current status. J Vasc Interv Radiol 2010;21:S242–50.

79. Dupuy DE, Liu D, Hartfeil D, et al. Percutaneous radiofrequency ablation of painful osseous metastases: a multicenter American College of Radiology Imaging Network trial. Cancer 2010;116:989–97.

80. Goetz MP, Callstrom MR, Charboneau JW, et al. Percutaneous image-guided radiofrequency ablation of painful metastases involving bone: a multicenter study. J Clin Oncol 2004;22:300–6.

81. Callstrom MR, Atwell TD, Charboneau JW, et al. Painful metastases involving bone: percutaneous image-guided croablation—prospective trial interim analysis. Radiology 2006;241:572–80.

82. Anselmetti GC, Manca A, Ortega C, et al. Treatment of extraspinal painful bone metastases with percutaneous cementoplasty: a prospective study of 50 patients. Cardiovasc Intervent Radiol 2008;31:1165–73.

83. Munk PL, Rashid F, Heran MK, et al. Combined cementoplasty and radiofrequency ablation in the treatment of painful neoplastic lesions of bone. J Vasc Interv Radiol 2009;20:903–11.

84. Barton PP, Waneck RE, Karnel FJ, et al. Embolization of bone metastases. J Vasc Interv Radiol 1996;7:81–8.

85. Forauer AR, Kent E, Cwikiel W, et al. Selective palliative transcatheter embolization of bony metastases from renal cell carcinoma. Acta Oncol 2007;46:1012–8.

86. Wang PJ, Shang MY, Qian Z, et al. CT-guided percutaneous neurolytic celiac plexus block technique. Abdom Imaging 2006;31:710–8.

87. Mercadante S, Nicosia F. Celiac plexus block: a reappraisal. Reg Anesth Pain Med 1998;23:37–48.

88. Reisfield GM, Wilson GR. Blocks of the sympathetic axis for visceral pain, 2nd edition. Fast Facts and Concepts #97. Available at: http://www.eperc.mcw.edu/fastFact/ff_97.htm. Accessed July 20, 2010.

89. Polati E, Finco G, Gottin L, et al. Prospective randomized double-blind trial of neurolytic celiac plexus block in patients with pancreatic cancer. Br J Surg 1998;85:199–201.

90. Becker G, Galandi D, Blum HE. Malignant ascites: systematic review and guideline for treatment. Eur J Cancer 2006;42:589–97.

91. McNamara P. Paracentesis – an effective method of symptom control in the palliative care setting? Palliat Med 2000;14:62–4.

92. Seike M, Maetani I, Saki Y. Treatment of malignant ascites in patients with advanced cancer: peritoneovenous shunt versus paracentesis. J Gastroenterol Hepatol 2007;22:2161–6.

93. Runyon BA. Refractory ascites. Semin Liver Dis 1993;13:343–51.

94. Runyon B, Montano A, Akriviadis A, et al. The serum-ascites albumin gradient is superior to the exudates-transudate concept in the differential diagnosis of ascites. Ann Intern Med 1992;117:215–20.

95. Hou W, Sanyal AJ. Ascites: diagnosis and management. Med Clin North Am 2009;93:801–17.

96. Husbands EL. Targeting diuretic use for malignant ascites. Two case reports highlighting the value of the serum-ascites albumin gradient in a palliative setting. J Pain Symptom Manage 2010;39:e7–9.

97. Pockros PJ, Esrason KT, Nguyen C, et al. Mobilization of malignant ascites with diuretics is dependant on ascetic fluid characteristics. Gastroenterology 1992; 103:1302–6.

98. D'Amico G, Luca A, Morabito A, et al. Uncovered transjugular introhepatic portosystemic shunt for refractory ascites: a meta-analysis. Gastroenterology 2005; 129:1282–93.

99. Rössle M, Ochs A, Gülberg V, et al. A comparison of paracentesis and transjugular intrahepatic portosystemic shunting in patients with ascites. N Engl J Med 2000;342:1701–7.

100. Salerno F, Merli M, Riggio O, et al. Randomized controlled study of TIPS versus paracentesis plus albumin in cirrhosis with severe ascites. Hepatology 2004;40: 629–35.

101. Salerno F, Camma C, Enea M, et al. Transjugular intrahepatic portosystemic shunt for refractory ascites: a meta-analysis of individual patient data. Gastroenterology 2007;133:825–34.

102. Kalva SP, Salazar GM, Walker TG. Transjugular intrahepatic portosystemic shunt for acute variceal hemorrhage. Tech Vasc Interv Radiol 2009;12:92–101.

103. Harrod-Kim P, Saad W, Waldman D. Predictors of early mortality after transjugular intrahepatic portosystemic shunt creation for the treatment of refractory ascites. J Vasc Interv Radiol 2006;17:1605–10.105.

104. Adam RA, Adam YG. Malignant ascites: past, present, and future. J Am Coll Surg 2004;198:999–1011.

105. Cheung DK, Raaf JH. Selection of patients with malignant ascites for peritoneovenous shunt. Cancer 1982;50:1204–9.

106. Campbell C. Controlling malignant ascites. Eur J Palliat Care 2001;8:187–9.

107. Runyon BA. Care of patients with ascites. N Engl J Med 1994;330:337–42.

108. Ringenberg QS, Doll DC, Loy TS, et al. Malignant ascites of unknown origin. Cancer 1989;64:753–5.

109. Spratt JS, Edwards M, Kubota T, et al. Peritoneal carcinomatosis: anatomy, physiology, diagnosis, management. Curr Probl Cancer 1986;10:558–84.

110. Coates G, Bush RS, Aspin N. A study of ascites using lymphoscintigraphy with 99 m Tc-sulfur colloid. Radiology 1973;107:577–83.

111. Beecham JB, Kucera P, HelmKamp BF, et al. Peritoneal angiogenesis in patients with ascites. Gynecol Oncol 1983;15:142.

112. Senger DR, Galli SJ, Dvorrak AM, et al. Tumor cells secrete a vascular permeability factor that promotes accumulation of ascites fluid. Science 1983;219:983–5.

113. Garrison RN, Vaclin LD, Galloway RH, et al. Malignant ascites. Clinical and experimental observations. Ann Surg 1986;203:644–51.

114. Parsons SL, Watson SA, Steele RJC. Malignant ascites. Br J Surg 1996;83:6–14.

115. Tarin D, Price JE, Kettlewell MG, et al. Cinicopathological observations on metastasis in man studied in patients treated with peritoneovenous shunts. Br Med J 1984;288:749–51.

116. Courtney A, Nemcek AA, Rosenberg S, et al. Prospective evaluation of the PleurX catheter when used to treat recurrent ascites associated with malignancy. J Vasc Interv Radiol 2008;19:1723–31.

117. Shields TW. Parapneumonic empyema. In: Shields TW, editor. General thoracic surgery. 4th edition. Baltimore (MD): Williams & Wilkins; 1994. p. 684–93.

118. Molnar TF. Current surgical treatment of thoracic empyema in adults. Eur J Cardiothorac Surg 2007;32:422–30.

119. Mahmoud TA, Ismail NI, Muda AS, et al. Bismuth paste injection for empyema thoracis: a 100-year-old method revisited. Ann Thorac Surg 2010;90:654–5.

120. Pollak JS, Burdge CM, Rosenblatt M, et al. Treatment of malignant pleural effusions with tunneled long-term drainage catheters. J Vasc Interv Radiol 2001;12: 201–8.

121. Aydogmus U, Ozdemir S, Cansever L, et al. Bedside talc pleurodesis for malignant pleural effusion: factors affecting success. Ann Surg Oncol 2009;16: 745–50.

122. Lombardi G, Zustovich F, Nicoletto MO, et al. Diagnosis and treatment of malignant pleural effusion: a systematic literature review and new approaches. Am J Clin Oncol 2010;33:420–3.

123. Ozyurtkan MO, Balci AE, Cakmak M. Predictors of mortality within three months in the patients with malignant pleural effusion. Eur J Intern Med 2010;21:30–4.

124. Davies HE, Lee YC, Davies RJ. Pleurodesis for malignant pleural effusion: talc, toxicity and where next? Thorax 2008;63:572–4.

125. Maskell NA, Lee YC, Gleeson FV, et al. Randomized trials describing lung inflammation after pleurodesis with talc of varying particle size. Am J Respir Crit Care Med 2004;170:377–82.

126. Ferrer J, Montes JF, Villarino MA, et al. Influence of particle size on extrapleural talc dissemination after talc slurry pleurodesis. Chest 2002;122:1018–27.

127. Dresler CM, Olak J, Herndon JE, et al. Phase III intergroup study of talc poudrage vs talc slurry sclerosis for malignant pleural effusion. Chest 2005;127: 909–15.

128. Janssen JP, Collier G, Astoul P, et al. Safety of pleurodesis with talc poudrage in malignant pleural effusion: a prospective cohort study. Lancet 2007; 369:1535–9.

129. Olden AM, Holloway R. Treatment of malignant pleural effusion: PleuRx catheter or talc pleurodesis? A cost-effectiveness analysis. J Palliat Med 2010;13:59–65.

130. El-Serag HB. Hepatocellular carcinoma: recent trends in the United States. Gastroenterology 2004;127:S27–34.

131. Dhanasekaran R, Khanna V, Kooby DA, et al. The effectiveness of locoregional therapies versus supportive care in maintaining survival within the Milan Criteria in patients with hepatocellular carcinoma. J Vasc Interv Radiol 2010;21: 1197–204.

132. Mazzaferro V, Chun YS, Poon RT, et al. Liver transplantation for hepatocellular carcinoma. Ann Surg Oncol 2008;15:1001–7.

133. McWilliams JP, Yamamoto S, Raman SS, et al. Percutaneous ablation of hepatocellular carcinoma: current status. J Vasc Interv Radiol 2010;21:S204–13.

134. Chen MS, Li JQ, Zheng Y, et al. A prospective randomized trial comparing percutaneous local ablative therapy and partial hepatectomy for small hepatocellular carcinoma. Ann Surg 2006;243:321–8.

135. Lü MD, Kuang M, Liang LJ, et al. Surgical resection versus percutaneous thermal ablation for early-stage hepatocellular carcinoma: a randomized clinical trial. Zhonghua Yi Xue Za Zhi 2006;86:801–5 [in Chinese].

136. Hong SN, Lee SY, Choi MS, et al. Comparing the outcomes of radiofrequency ablation and surgery in patients with a single small hepatocellular carcinoma and well-preserved hepatic hunction. J Clin Gastroenterol 2005;39:247–52.

137. Lupo L, Panzera P, Giannelli G, et al. Single hepatocellular carcinoma ranging from 3 to 5 cm: radiofrequency ablation or resection? HPB(Oxford) 2007;9: 429–34.

138. Montorsi M, Santambrogio R, Bianchi P, et al. Survival and recurrences after hepatic resection or radiofrequency for hepatocellular carcinoma in cirrhotic patients: a multivariate analysis. J Gastrointest Surg 2005;9:62–7.

139. Ren ZG, Gan YH, Fan J, et al. Treatment of postoperative recurrence of hepato-cellular carcinoma with radiofrequency ablation comparing with repeated surgical resection. Zhonghua Wai Ke Za Zhi 2008;46:1614–6 [in Chinese].

140. Lencioni RA, Allgaier HP, Cioni D, et al. Small hepatocellular carcinoma in cirrhosis: randomized comparison of radio-frequency thermal ablation versus percutaneous ethanol injection. Radiology 2003;228:235–40.

141. Brunello F, Veltri A, Carucci P, et al. Radiofrequency ablation versus ethanol injection for early hepatocellular carcinoma: a randomized controlled trial. Scand J Gastroenterol 2008;43:727–35.

142. Zhang YJ, Liang HH, Chen MS, et al. Hepatocellular carcinoma treated with radiofrequency ablation with or without ethanol injection: a prospective random-ized trial. Radiology 2007;244:599–607.

143. Kwan SW, Kerlan RK, Sunshine JH. Utilization of interventional oncology treat-ments in the United States. J Vasc Interv Radiol 2010;21:1054–60.

144. Massarweh NN, Park JO, Farjah F, et al. Trands in the utilization and impact of radiofrequency ablation for hepatocellular carcinoma. J Am Coll Surg 2010; 210:441–8.

145. Gervais DA, Goldberg SN, Brown DB, et al. Society of Interventional Radiology position statement on percutaneous radiofrequency ablation for the treatment of liver tumors. J Vasc Interv Radiol 2009;20:3–8.

146. Brown DB, Geschwind JFH, Soulen MC, et al. Society of interventional radiology position statement on chemoembolization of hepatic malignancies. J Vasc Interv Radiol 2009;20:S317–23.

147. Brown DB, Cardella JF, Sacks D, et al. Quality improvement guidelines for trans-hepatic arterial chemoembization, embolization, and chemotherapeutic infusion for hepatic malignancy. J Vasc Interv Radiol 2009;20:S219–26.

148. Miyayama S, Yamashiro M, Okuda M, et al. Chemoembolization for the treat-ment of large hepatocellular carcinoma. J Vasc Interv Radiol 2010;21: 1226–34.

149. Brown DB, Fundakowski CE, Lisker-Melman M, et al. Comparison of MELD and Child-Pugh scores to predict survival after chemoembolization for hepatocellular carcinoma. J Vasc Interv Radiol 2004;15:1209–18.

150. Lo C, Ngan H, Tso W, et al. Randomized controlled trial of transarterial lipiodol chemoembolization for unresectable hepatocellular carcinoma. Hepatology 2002;35:1164–71.

151. Salem R, Lewandowski RJ, Atassi B, et al. Treatment of unresectable hepatocel-lular carcinoma with use of 90Y microspheres (TheraSphere): safety, tumor response, and survival. J Vasc Interv Radiol 2005;16:1627–39.

152. Stuart K, Stokes K, Jenkins R, et al. Treatment of hepatocellular carcinoma using doxorubicin/ethiodized oil/gelatin powder chemoembolization. Cancer 1993;72: 3202–9.

153. Berger DH, Carrasco CH, Hohn DC, et al. Hepatic artery chemoembolization or embolization for primary and metastatic liver tumors: post-treatment manage-ment and complications. J Surg Oncol 1995;60:116–21.

154. Kennedy A, Nag S, Salem R, et al. Recommendations for radioembolization of hepatic malignancies using yttrium-90 microsphere brachytherapy: a consensus panel report from the Radioembolization Brachytherapy Oncology Consortium. Int J Radiat Oncol Biol Phys 2007;68:13–23.

155. Goin JE, Salem R, Carr BI, et al. Treatment of unresectable hepatocellular carci-noma with intrahepatic yttrium 90 microspheres: a risk-stratification analysis. J Vasc Interv Radiol 2005;16:195–203.

156. Sasson AR, Sigurdson ER. Surgical treatment of liver metastases. Semin Oncol 2002;29:107–18.

157. Jaffe BM, Donegan WL, Watson F, et al. Factors influencing survival in patients with untreated hepatic metastases. Surg Gynecol Obstet 1968;127:1–11.

158. Bramhall SR, Gur U, Coldham C, et al. Liver resection for colorectal metastases. Ann R Coll Surg Engl 2003;85:334–9.

159. Smith MD, McCall JL. Systematic review of tumour number and outcome after radical treatment of colorectal liver metastases. Br J Surg 2009;96:1101–13.

160. Dimick JB, Cowan JA, Knol JA, et al. Hepatic resection in the United States: indications, outcomes, and hospital procedural volumes from a nationally representative database. Arch Surg 2003;138:185–91.

161. Gazelle GS, Hunink M, Kuntz KM, et al. Cost-effectiveness of hepatic metastasectomy in patients with metastatic colorectal carcinoma: a state-transition Monte Carlo decision analysis. Ann Surg 2003;237:544–55.

162. Nordlinger B, Van Cutsem E, Rougier P, et al. Does chemotherapy prior to liver resection increase the potential for cure in patients with metastatic colorectal cancer? A report from the European Colorectal Metastases Treatment Group. Eur J Cancer 2007;43:2037–45.

163. Nicolay NH, Berry DP, Sharma RA. Liver metastases from colorectal cancer: radioembolization with systemic therapy. Nat Rev Clin Oncol 2009;6:687–97.

164. Mulier S, Ruers T, Jamart J, et al. Radiofrequency ablation versus resection for resectable colorectal liver metastases: time for a randomized trial? An update. Dig Surg 2008;25:445–60.

165. Wong SL, Mangu PB, Choti MA, et al. American Society of Clinical Oncology 2009 clinical evidence review on radiofrequency ablation of hepatic metastases from colorectal cancer. J Clin Oncol 2009;28:493–508.

166. Solbiati L, Livraghi T, Goldberg SN, et al. Percutaneous radio-frequency ablation of hepatic metastases from colorectal cancer: long-term results in 117 patients. Radiology 2001;221:159–66.

167. Livraghi T, Solbiati L, Meloni F, et al. Percutaneous radiofrequency ablation of liver metastases in potential candidates for resection: the "test-of-time" approach. Cancer 2003;97:3027–35.

168. Abdalla EK, Vauthey JN, Ellis LM, et al. Recurrence and outcomes following hepatic resection, radiofrequency ablation, and combined resection/ablation for colorectal liver metasteses. Ann Surg 2004;239:818–25.

169. Amersi FF, McElrath-Garza A, Ahmad A, et al. Long-term survival after radiofrequency ablation of complex unresectable liver tumors. Arch Surg 2006;141:581–7.

170. Chow DH, Sinn FM, Ng KK, et al. Radiofrequency ablation for hepatocellular carcinoma and metastatic liver tumors: a comparative study. J Surg Oncol 2006;94:565–71.

171. Kuvshinoff BW, Ota DM. Radiofrequency ablation of liver tumors: influence of technique and tumor size. Surgery 2002;132:605–11.

172. Sanz-Altamira PM, Spence LD, Huberman MS, et al. Selective chemoembolization in the management of hepatic metastases in refractory colorectal carcinoma: a phase II trial. Dis Colon Rectum 1997;40:770–5.

173. Soulen MC. Chemoembolization of hepatic malignancies. Semin Intervent Radiol 1997;14:305–11.

174. Gray BN, Burton MA, Kelleher DK, et al. Selective internal radiation (SIR) therapy for treatment of liver metastases: measurement of response rate. J Surg Oncol 1989;42:192–6.

175. Gray BN, Anderson JE, Burton MA, et al. Regression of liver metastases following treatment with yttrium-90 microspheres. Aust N Z J Surg 1992;62: 105–10.

176. Stubbs RS, Cannan RJ, Mitchell AW. Selective internal radiation therapy (SIRT) with 90Yttrium microspheres for extensive colorectal liver metastases. Hepato-gastroenterology 2001;48:333–7.

177. Jakobs TF, Hoffmann RT, Dehm K, et al. Hepatic yttrium-90 radioembolization of chemotherapy-refractory colorectal cancer liver metastases. J Vasc Interv Radiol 2008;19:1187–95.

178. Gray B, Van Hazel G, Hope M, et al. Randomised trial of SIR-Spheres plus chemotherapy vs. chemotherapy alone for treating patients with liver metastases from primary large bowel cancer. Ann Oncol 2001;12:1711–20.

179. Van Hazel G, Blackwell A, Anderson J, et al. Randomised phase 2 trial of SIR-Spheres plus fluorouracil/leucovorin chemotherapy versus fluorouracil/leucovorin chemotherapy alone in advanced colorectal cancer. J Surg Oncol 2004;88:78–85.

Palliative Care in Lung Cancer

Betty Ferrell, PhD, RN, MA[a],*, Marianna Koczywas, MD[b],
Fred Grannis, MD[c], Annie Harrington, MD[d]

KEYWORDS

• Palliative care • Quality of life • Symptom management

An estimated 222,000 new cases of lung cancer were diagnosed in the United States in 2010, and approximately 157,000 patients died from the disease.[1] Despite complete resection and curative intent, many patients with early stage, resectable lung cancer experience recurrence. After potentially curative surgical resection, the 5-year survival rate for early stage non–small cell lung carcinoma (NSCLC) is commonly accepted to be 60% to 80% for stage I, 40% to 50% for stage II, and 10% to 20% for stage IIIA.[2,3] Two thirds of these patients recur systemically, and the remaining one third recur locally.[4] Because recurrent disease is common, aggressive symptom management and support using an interdisciplinary palliative care model becomes an important aspect of care. This article describes the role of palliative care for patients with lung cancer.

DEFINING PALLIATIVE CARE

Palliative care is a concept in medical care that has expanded within the last decade to address the supportive care needs that accompany the occurrence of life-threatening disease. The concept addresses different aspects in the trajectory of cancer. In its recent 2009 update, the National Consensus Project Clinical Practice Guidelines for Quality Palliative Care defines palliative care as "medical care provided by an interdisciplinary team, including the professions of medicine, nursing, social work, chaplaincy, counseling, nursing assistant, and other health care professions focused on the relief of suffering and support for the best possible quality of life (QOL) for patients facing

This work is supported by Grant No. P01-CA136396–01 from the National Cancer Institute.
The authors have nothing to disclose.
[a] Department of Population Sciences, Nursing Research and Education, City of Hope, 1500 East Duarte Road, Duarte, CA 91010, USA
[b] Division of Medical Oncology and Therapeutics Research, Thoracic Oncology and Lung Cancer Program, City of Hope, 1500 East Duarte Road, Duarte, CA 91010, USA
[c] Department of Surgery, Thoracic Cancer Program, City of Hope, 1500 East Duarte Road, Duarte, CA 91010, USA
[d] Department of Medicine, Division of Pulmonary and Critical Care, Cedars Sinai Medical Center, 8700 Beverly Boulevard, Room 6732, Los Angeles, CA 90048, USA
* Corresponding author.
E-mail address: bferrell@coh.org

serious life-threatening illness and their families. It aims to identify and address the physical, psychological, spiritual, and practical burdens of illness". **Fig. 1** illustrates how palliative care fits with the treatment of lung cancer.[5] Palliative care begins at the time of diagnosis of a serious disease; continues throughout treatment, cure, or until death; and involves the family during the bereavement period.

Studies have been conducted during the past few decades to determine the effect of early introduction of palliative care in cancer. Recently, Temel and colleagues[6] published findings from a randomized clinical trial to examine the effect of introducing palliative care at diagnosis on QOL changes at 12 weeks for patients with metastatic NSCLC. Patients enrolled in the study received either early palliative care integrated with standard oncologic care or standard oncologic care alone (N = 151). Results were in favor of the early palliative care group, where better QOL was observed compared with patients who received only standard oncologic care. Fewer depressive symptoms were observed for the palliative care group. Most interestingly, patients in the palliative care group received less aggressive care at the end of life, but their median survival was longer (11.6 months vs 8.9 months; $P = .02$).[6]

QOL and Symptoms in Early Stage NSCLC

Several studies have described QOL in early stage NSCLC postoperatively. Balduyck and colleagues[7] followed 100 patients with NSCLC for 12 months postoperatively and found that the QOL evolution in patients who received a lobectomy or wedge resection was comparable with a 1-month transient decrease in functioning and increase in pain. Other studies have found similar transient QOL decreases postoperatively, with general recovery seen between 3 and 9 months postoperatively.[8,9] Patients who underwent a pneumonectomy had the worst outcome, with poor physical functioning, poor role functioning, pain, dyspnea, emotional problems, and decreased pulmonary functions that did not recover to baseline.[10] Pneumonectomy was also found to be predictive for hospital readmissions and mortality postoperatively.[11]

In a longitudinal study exploring QOL in patients with resected NSCLC 2 years postoperatively, surgery substantially reduced QOL across all dimensions except emotional functioning.[4] Approximately half of patients continued to experience symptoms and diminished functioning after 2 years.[12] In a study with long-term survivors of lung cancer (>5 years), Sarna and colleagues[13] found that 22% of survivors had distressed mood, and 50% experienced moderate to severe pulmonary distress.

Studies have also identified determinants of QOL after pulmonary resections. Preoperative QOL has been found to predict postoperative QOL, with continued declines in physical, social, and psychological states and slower recovery.[12,13] Factors that provoke the most fear in patients with resectable NSCLC are not surgical risks of perioperative morbidity or mortality, but the physical and mental handicaps that hinder recovery postoperatively.[14,15] Common disease and treatment-related symptoms include dyspnea, cough, fatigue, pain, lack of appetite, and insomnia.[16]

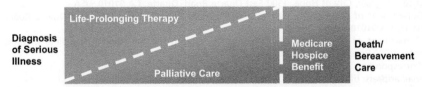

Fig. 1. How palliative care fits with the treatment of lung cancer. Palliative care begins at the time of diagnosis of a serious disease; continues throughout treatment, cure, or until death; and involves the family during the bereavement period.

The average number of symptoms per patient in NSCLC has been reported to be around 14 with 2.3 symptoms rated as severe.[17]

In a systematic review of symptoms in lung cancer, Cooley[16] concluded that patients with lung cancer experienced multiple symptoms that differed across illness trajectories and treatments. In early stage NSCLC where surgical interventions are the primary treatment, postoperative symptoms include pain and dyspnea.[3] Postthoracotomy pain syndrome is defined as an aching or burning sensation that persists or recurs along the thoracotomy scar at least 2 months postoperatively, and neuropathic symptoms, such as paresthesia–dysesthesia and hypoesthesia, are reported in 69% and 40% of patients, respectively.[18,19] Immediately after a thoracotomy, 90% of patients report varying degrees of pain.[20] The incidence of chronic postthoracotomy pain is estimated to be 26% to 67%.[20] Predictors of chronic postthoracotomy pain include severe acute postoperative pain, high consumption of analgesics postoperatively, female gender, the extent of surgery, and psychological distress.[21,22]

Respiratory symptoms, such as cough, dyspnea, wheeze, and hemoptysis, are common in NSCLC, occurring in 40% to 85% of patients.[23] These symptoms may be present at diagnosis or as a direct result of treatment, and prevalence is dependent on tumor type, disease stage, gender, age, and living situations.[24,25] Dales and colleagues[26] followed patients with NSCLC after thoracic surgery and found that dyspnea and QOL deteriorated up to 3 months postoperatively, but returned to baseline at 9 months. In a study exploring dyspnea and QOL in patients with both early and late stage NSCLC (N = 120), Smith and colleagues[25] found that advanced disease was not correlated with dyspnea. This finding suggests that patients with early stage NSCLC who are most likely to be cured may also be faced with debilitating breathlessness that results in poor QOL during survivorship.[27,28] In one large prospective cohort study of 939 patients with stage III or IV NSCLC hospitalized at five teaching hospitals in the United States, severe dyspnea was recorded in 32% of patients, and in 90% of patients near death.[29]

The psychological implications of lung cancer have been documented extensively in the literature. A number of studies have documented the presence of depression among patients with lung cancer, with an incidence rate of 15% to 44% in patients with newly diagnosed NSCLC.[30] Studies have shown that the 1-, 2-, and 3-month prevalence of depression in patients with NSCLC after curative resection was 9%, 9.4%, and 5.8%, respectively.[31] The prevalence of psychological distress is the highest among patients with lung cancer compared with solid tumors.[19] Factors that are associated with psychological distress include such symptoms as pain, poor performance, age, social support, physician support, and marital status.[19] Faller and Bulzebruck[32] studied coping and survival in 103 patients with lung cancer using a 10-year follow-up. Coping was assessed before treatment by using both self-reports and interviewer ratings. Findings suggest that self-reported depressive coping style was linked with shorter survival, and active coping style was linked with longer survival. Maliski and colleagues[33] interviewed 29 lung cancer survivors (>10 years) and identified five key themes: (1) existential issues, (2) health and self-care, (3) physical ability, (4) adjustment, and (5) support.

Research has shown that social support is associated with distress among patients with cancer and is positively related to QOL.[34,35] Walker and colleagues[36] found that the type of social support available to patients with NSCLC predicted more adaptive coping in early stage disease (N = 119). A more assisting and cooperative support that leaves responsibilities and choices to the patient was associated with adaptive coping, whereas support that entails others taking responsibility for tasks and telling the patient what to do was associated with less adaptive coping.[36] Worries about the illness, family, and the future relating to the illness are the most common psychosocial concerns.[37] Hill and colleagues[37] reported that less than half of the concerns of patients with NSCLC (43%) were discussed by providers. Patients' psychosocial symptoms were more worrisome than physical symptoms, and psychosocial concerns were least likely to have been dealt with effectively.[37]

Diagnosis of a life-threatening disease, such as NSCLC, can cause enormous spiritual distress. Finding meaning in illness has shown to positively affect QOL. A cross-sectional study conducted by Downe-Wamboldt and colleagues[38] documented that overall QOL in patients with NSCLC is predicted most by meaning of illness, specifically the illness being perceived as manageable. In a study conducted among 60 patients with NSCLC, Meraviglia[39] found that people who reported more meaning in life had better psychological well-being. Furthermore, as the level of meaning in life increased, symptom distress decreased among the study participants. Finally, Sarna and colleagues[40] examined the relationship between meaning of illness and QOL in women with NSCLC (N = 217). Findings suggest that depressed mood, negative conceptualizations of meaning of illness, and younger age explained 37% of the variance of global QOL and were correlated with poorer QOL. In this study, more than a third of patients associated lung cancer with negative meaning.[40]

Palliative Symptom Management in Lung Cancer

Given the multitude of symptoms patients can experience, alleviating discomfort often requires several treatment modalities to reach an acceptable goal of palliation. With respect to decrements in QOL related specifically to the tumor itself, the general assault on health by lung cancer can be broadly separated into four categories of clinical problems: (1) those caused by the primary tumor, (2) those caused by metastases, (3) those caused by treatment, and (4) those caused by paraneoplastic syndromes.[41] In addition to problems attributable to the diagnosis of lung cancer, patients also often carry the burden of significant comorbid disease. Because the average age of presentation of lung cancer is 71,[42] a sizable percentage of patients with lung cancer have preexisting disease, both related and unrelated to tobacco products. Such tobacco-related diseases include cerebrovascular disease, coronary vascular disease, peripheral vascular disease, heart failure, aortic aneurysm, and chronic obstructive pulmonary disease (COPD). Despite the presence of these multiple comorbid diseases, most patients with lung cancer die of the lung cancer rather than the comorbid diseases, even when lung cancer presents in early stage.

Symptom management begins with a conversation between provider and patient, taking time to assess the patient's symptoms and educate the patient and family about possible treatment options. Clinicians should evaluate for potentially correctable causes of discomfort, and proceed with noninterventional symptom management if no cause can be identified.[41] An awareness of the multiple treatment modalities available for palliation of symptoms related to lung cancer can aid the clinician in obtaining timely relief for the patient, who may have very little time remaining.

Palliative Surgical Options

The most common clinical situations in patients with lung cancer that may benefit from invasive interventions include airway obstruction, hemoptysis, pleural or pericardial effusions, and brain or bone metastases. Worsening symptoms of dyspnea, hemoptysis, and stridor warrant prompt bronchoscopic evaluation for airway obstruction. Airway obstruction can be inside the airway, within the airway wall, or extrinsically compressing the airway.[43,44] Palliative bronchoscopy with the goal of alleviating symptoms can be highly effective. Bronchoscopic options for treatment include short-term endotracheal intubation, tumor debulking, balloon dilation, laser therapy, electrocautery, cryotherapy, photodynamic therapy, argon plasma coagulation, and airway stent placement.[45] Airway obstruction can be endobronchial or extrinsic compression. When malignant central airway obstruction resulted in respiratory failure, urgent therapeutic bronchoscopy allowed 52% of patients to come off the ventilator in one study.[46] Balloon dilation is best used in conjunction with stent placement, and works best when small areas are stenosed.[47] Laser debridement and electrocautery are only effective for intraluminal lesions, but can result in immediate relief of dyspnea in 55% to 90% of patients.[48,49] Cryotherapy and photodynamic therapy are also highly effective in relieving symptoms caused by intraluminal airway obstruction, but require repeat treatment sessions with slow symptom relief.[50]

Airway stents can be used for both intrinsic and extrinsic compressing lesions, and can be used in conjunction with other techniques including balloon dilation and laser debridement. The only true contraindication to stent placement is external airway compression by a vessel, because this can result in high rates of erosion, hemorrhage, and death.[51] Airway stents are also sometimes considered for palliative management of tracheoesophageal fistulas. Tracheoesophageal fistulas carry significant symptom burden for patients (ie, aspiration or pneumonitis), along with inability to tolerate oral intake and marked reduced survival of 1 to 7 weeks.[41] Aggressive interventions, such as attempts at surgical repair or resection, should be avoided, and stenting of both trachea and esophagus has yielded only modest benefit in limited trials.[52–55] One small study of 24 patients showed that invasive treatment of endobronchial obstruction resulted in improved airway diameter in all patients and improved dyspnea in 85% of patients, but failed to show a significant improvement in QOL scores.[56]

Massive hemoptysis can be very distressing to patients, families, and physicians, and prompt bronchoscopic evaluation for possible palliative therapy can be of benefit in some cases. Hemoptysis is a second clinical scenario in which invasive procedures may palliate symptoms of lung cancer. Although physicians often define massive hemoptysis warranting intervention as greater than 200 mL in 24 hours, patients often consider small amounts of hemoptysis very concerning.[57] Otherwise healthy persons presenting with hemoptysis are candidates for open lung surgery; however, patients with lung cancer with hemoptysis often have advanced disease, which makes them poor surgical candidates, and thus may benefit from less aggressive interventions. Therapeutic bronchoscopy with balloon tamponade and infusion of vasoactive agents, such as epinephrine, may be successful as a temporizing measure.[58–62] If the area of bleeding can be directly visualized, bronchoscopic techniques, such as neodymium:yttrium-aluminum-garnet laser coagulation or electrocautery can also be used, with reported response rates of 60% to 100%.[63–65] Bronchial angiography with bronchial artery embolization can sometimes control hemoptysis.

Malignant pleural and pericardial effusions are a third common cause of dyspnea in patients with lung cancer that can also be treated with palliative interventional procedures. When a pleural effusion is found in a patients with lung cancer presenting with dyspnea, a diagnostic thoracentesis should first be done. The initial thoracentesis helps to determine if drainage relieves the patient's dyspnea and allows the lung to fully reexpand. For those with malignant pleural effusions and symptomatic improvement after thoracentesis, the recommended therapeutic options include serial thoracenteses, chest tube drainage with bedside chemical pleurodesis, surgical pleurodesis, or pleural drain catheter placement.

Repeat thoracentesis is recommended in patients with very short life expectancy, because malignant pleural effusions recur in nearly 100% of patients within 1 month of initial drainage.[40] Chemical pleurodesis carries a 50% to 95% success rate, and seems to be most successful when performed using talc, according to a recent

Cochran review.[66] Chemical pleurodesis can be done at the bedside but requires chest tube placement and a prolonged hospital stay; it can also occasionally be painful and cause pneumonitis in 4% to 8% of patients.[67] Surgical pleurodesis is slightly more successful with a 75% to 100% success rate,[41] but many patients with advanced lung cancer are unlikely to be fit surgical candidates. Chemical pleurodesis requires an expanded lung for success, and in patients who have rapidly accumulating effusions with trapped lung, these techniques are more likely to fail.

Tunneled pleural catheters have been recommended as first line for malignant pleural effusions, because they can be done as an outpatient, require only local anesthesia, and have high success rates of 85% to 95%. In 1999, Putnam and colleagues[68] conducted a trial that led to Food and Drug Administration approval of the PleurX catheter (CareFusion, San Diego, CA, USA), showing that pleurodesis with doxycycline had an average hospital stay of 6.5 days, whereas tunneled PleurX catheter placement required only 1 day.

In a recent paper advocating for tunneled pleural catheter placement as first-line treatment of malignant pleural effusions, Tremblay and colleagues[69] wrote, "the current authors estimate that 1 week in the hospital represents 5% of a patient's remaining life expectancy, time that may be more beneficial spent at home with family and friends." Recent cost-effectiveness analysis showed that tunneled pleural catheters became more cost effective when the life expectancy was 6 weeks or less.[70] The study did not account for physician inpatient fees in the pleurodesis group and assumed three nursing visits per week were needed for the indwelling catheter group; given that the patient and family can easily be taught to care for the catheter and physician fees can be costly, the cost benefit of tunneled catheters is probably more pronounced than stated.

A review of 231 catheters placed for malignant pleural effusions showed a low infection rate of 2.2%, usually limited to local cellulitis, and confirmed a high effectiveness rate, with 52 of 52 catheters placed for lung cancer still in place and functional at the time of death.[67] Malignant pleural effusions are a treatable cause of dyspnea in patients with lung cancer, and the selection of treatment method should be based on minimizing patient burden while maximizing symptom improvement and QOL.

Superior vena cava syndrome occurs in 10% of patients with lung cancer involving the right hilum.[71] Obstruction leads to a characteristic syndrome, with formation of collateral veins over the upper chest, facial swelling made worse with recumbency, headache, increased cerebral venous pressure, and in severe cases blindness and coma. Palliation of these symptoms can often be achieved with a combination of chemotherapy and radiation therapy for NSCLC.

Surgical palliation with bypass of the cava has been uncommonly performed in highly selected circumstances, but more recently endovascular stent placement by interventional radiologists has had increased success at alleviating symptoms. Case series report success rates of 94% to 95% after stent placement, and many authors advocate stent placement as the initial treatment for immediate symptom relief with fewer complication.[72–84] Although surgery is the only curative treatment approach for lung cancer, the surgeon and interventional radiologist should be considered members of the extended team for the palliation of lung cancer symptoms.

Palliative Pharmacologic Options

Medications are invariably used in the management of pain and dyspnea in patients with lung cancer. Effective pain management may not mean complete pain relief, but more likely a significant alleviation in the patient's pain by at least 33% to 50%.[85–87] Pain medications should be administered in accordance with the National

Comprehensive Cancer Network Pain Guidelines,[88] beginning with nonopioids, such as nonsteroidal anti-inflammatory drugs and acetaminophen, and continuing with the addition of opioids and adjuvants as needed. When opioids are administered, constipation should be prophylaxed against and continuously monitored. For neuropathic pain, adjuvants to analgesics, such as anticonvulsants and tricyclic antidepressants, can be very helpful. Steroids can aid in relief of symptoms caused by edema from spinal and intracranial metastases, whereas bisphosphonates can reduce pain caused by bony metastases.[89] The medication regimen should be kept as simple as possible to avoid further side effect and cost burden. The oral route of administration is preferred. When this is not possible, rectal or transdermal delivery is often feasible. For parenterally administered medication, the intravenous or subcutaneous routes should be used. Intramuscular administration has the disadvantages of increased pain with administration and unpredictable absorption. Inhaled administration of opioids is not recommended.[90]

Dyspnea in the setting of lung cancer can be attributed to five causes: (1) direct involvement of lung tissue by cancer; (2) indirect respiratory complications related to the cancer (postobstructive pneumonia and pleural effusions); (3) treatment-related complications (fibrosis secondary to chemotherapy or radiation); (4) respiratory comorbidities (pulmonary embolism); and (5) other comorbid conditions (COPD, malnutrition, and prior lung resection).[41] Pharmacologic management options include bronchodilators, corticosteroids, anxiolytics, antidepressants, opioids, and oxygen. A metaanalysis of 18 randomized controlled trials confirmed that opioids are successful in relieving dyspnea.[91] Because many patients with lung cancer also have COPD, optimizing COPD treatment can be beneficial in relieving dyspnea. A prospective study of 100 terminally ill patients with cancer, 49 of whom had lung cancer, showed that correctable causes of dyspnea included bronchospasm in 52% of patients and hypoxia in 40% of patients.[92] Inhaled bronchodilators can assist with management of bronchospasm, whereas supplemental oxygen can treat dyspnea-related hypoxia. There is some debate as to whether oxygen can also alleviate dyspnea in patients who are nonhypoxemic; for the population with advanced lung cancer, oxygen prescription should be considered for all patients who are dyspneic regardless of oxygenation status, because it may improve exercise tolerance,[93] and should not be delayed awaiting painful serial blood gases to confirm hypoxemic status.

Cough is a complaint seen in the initial presentations of more than 65% of patients with lung cancer.[94] In addition to treatment for correctable causes of cough, pharmacologic therapies that may be of benefit include cough suppressants, bronchodilators, and opioids. Codeine is a popular and effective choice of opioid for suppressing this symptom. Medical management of comorbid conditions contributing to cough, such as COPD, gastroesophageal reflux, and congestive heart failure, can also be of benefit.[95]

When death is imminent, oral and respiratory secretions become salient symptoms. It is important to separate the nursing concerns of frequent suctioning, the family concerns of chest crackles, and the true symptoms of dyspnea or cough sensed by the patient. Although opioids are the most successful agents for management of dyspnea, anticholinergic agents, such as scopolamine and glycopyrrolate, are preferred for control of copious secretions. Such symptoms as pain and dyspnea that do not respond to initial therapy should prompt referral to palliative care and pain management specialists, from the time of presentation until the last days of life.

Palliative Chemotherapy

Palliative chemotherapy may increase survival, and in some cases can improve pain and other symptoms.[96-100] Palliative chemotherapy means chemotherapy given primarily for rapid relief of symptoms, not noncurative chemotherapy. Dyspnea related to pulmonary parenchymal toxicity from chemotherapy should be managed with discontinuation of the chemotherapeutic regimen and institution of steroids. This is a delicate balance in using chemotherapy to the full extent possible to relieve symptoms and reverse the underlying disease while also monitoring closely to determine when the chemotherapy may be adding to symptom burden and thus should be discontinued.[101]

Palliative Radiation

Palliative radiation therapy can be used throughout the course of lung cancer, before surgery, along with chemotherapy, or as an independent treatment modality. Radiation therapy can be used as primary treatment of a lung cancer in settings where surgery is not indicated, because of location of tumor, advanced stage, comorbidities, or patient preference. Radiation therapy can be of palliative benefit to alleviate pain and neurologic deficits from brain and spinal metastases, relieve pain from bone metastases, and prevention of impending pathologic fracture. Finally, radiation can also be given by way of interventional bronchoscopy as intraluminal brachytherapy to help control hemoptysis and airway obstruction by central tumors.

Radiation therapy has a wide spectrum of complications, depending on site, dose, method of dosing, and comorbid conditions. Although it is very uncommon for patients to die as a complication of radiation therapy, radiation pneumonitis can cause cough, shortness of breath, and even death in a small percentage of patients. Spontaneous rib fractures can occur after a radiation treatment of the chest. Radiation-induced mucositis, esophagitis, and skin changes are common complications, and the effect of radiation therapy on the heart and lung can combine with loss of function secondary to comorbid conditions and lung resection to impair cardiorespiratory function.[102]

Other Palliative Management Options

The broad term of "supportive care" for patients with advanced lung cancer can include a variety of medical, psychological, and alternative therapies, all of which can aid in the palliation of symptoms. One medical example is the use of blood transfusions, which can alleviate fatigue and dyspnea associated with anemia, and improve QOL.[103] Interventions, such as guided imagery, breathing techniques, and educational tools, can have a positive impact on common psychologic symptoms, such as anxiety and depression that undermine QOL. Finally, the involvement of social and spiritual support for patients and families cannot be underestimated, and can certainly impact physical symptoms and overall QOL. The task of integrating palliative surgical, medical, and psychosocial care for the management of a patient with advanced lung cancer requires an interdisciplinary team, with all members of the team focused on how best to provide relief of suffering and the best QOL possible for the patient's remaining years, days, or hours.

A Model for Integrating Palliative Care in Lung Cancer

Fig. 2 provides details on a model to improve palliative care for patients with lung cancer and their family caregivers. This model was developed based on extensive pilot work by the authors.[104,105] In our interdisciplinary palliative care model, a comprehensive assessment of patient and family caregivers' QOL concerns before treatment initiation begins this process of care. QOL assessment is focused on four domains: (1) physical, (2) psychological, (3) social, and (4) spiritual well-being. After the comprehensive QOL assessment, an interdisciplinary care team meeting is scheduled and

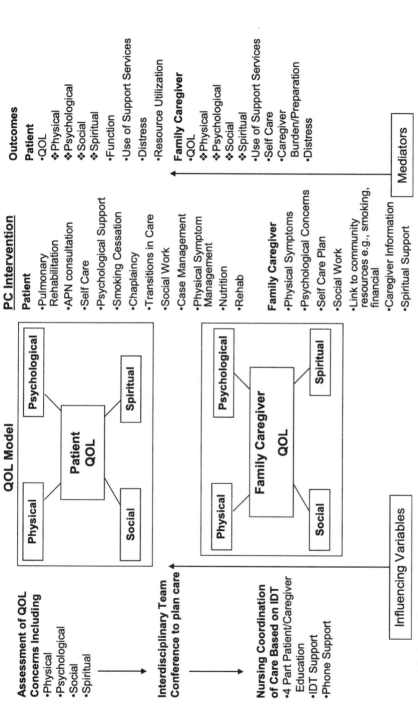

Fig. 2. A model of care for patients with lung cancer and family caregivers. APN, advance practice nurse; IDT, interdisciplinary team.

initiated. The team should include the patient's treating physicians; nurses involved in patient care; and supportive care experts, such as social workers, psychologists, spiritual counselors, pulmonary rehabilitation specialists, case managers, pain specialists, and dietitians. Together as an interdisciplinary team, the patient's QOL assessment, which includes physical, psychological, social, and spiritual dimensions, are discussed, and a care plan is produced to address each of the issues. Nursing coordination of care is initiated based on the recommendations of the team, and includes patient and caregiver education, support from the team members, and referrals to supportive care services. Patient and family caregiver outcomes to be measured should include QOL; functional status; use of support services; distress; use of resources; and family caregiver self-care, burden, and skills preparedness.

Initial pilot studies and the development of the model at the City of Hope led to the design of a 5-year program funded by the National Cancer Institute to test the effectiveness of the interdisciplinary palliative care model to improve care for patients with lung cancer and their family caregivers. Consistent with the recommendations of the Institute of Medicine Report on palliative care,[106] it is believed that palliative care, including symptom management and attention to QOL concerns of patients and families, should be addressed throughout the trajectory of lung cancer. Three simultaneous projects are included within the program project. Project 1 is early stage lung cancer, and provides a model of integrating palliative care throughout the trajectory of disease. Project 2 focuses on late-stage lung cancer, a population that has decreased survival and high QOL and symptom concerns. Project 3 focuses on family caregivers of patients with lung cancer.

SUMMARY

Lung cancer continues to be the second most common cancer in the United States with over 157,000 patients expected to die from the disease this year.[1] Advancements in the surgical and medical treatment of lung cancer have resulted in more favorable short-term survival outcomes. Treatment, however, can be complex, and long-term survival with the most current, cutting-edge technologies remains elusive. After initial treatment, lung cancer requires continued surveillance and follow-up for long-term side effects and possible recurrence. The integration of quality palliative care into routine clinical care of patients with lung cancer after surgical intervention is essential in preserving function and optimizing QOL through survivorship. An interdisciplinary palliative care model can effectively link patients to the appropriate supportive care services in a timely fashion.

REFERENCES

1. Jemal A, Siegel R, Xu J, et al. Cancer statistics, 2010. CA Cancer J Clin 2010; 60(5):277–300.
2. Scott WJ, Howington J, Feigenberg S, et al. Treatment of non-small cell lung cancer stage I and stage II: ACCP evidence-based clinical practice guidelines (2nd edition). Chest 2007;132(Suppl 3):234S–42S.
3. Spiro SG, Gould MK, Colice GL. Initial evaluation of the patient with lung cancer: symptoms, signs, laboratory tests, and paraneoplastic syndromes: ACCP evidenced-based clinical practice guidelines (2nd edition). Chest 2007; 132(Suppl 3):149S–60S.
4. Kenny PM, King MT, Viney RC, et al. Quality of life and survival in the 2 years after surgery for non small-cell lung cancer. J Clin Oncol 2008;26(2):233–41.

5. National Consensus Project. Clinical practice guidelines for quality palliative care 2009. Available at: www.nationalconsensusproject.org. Accessed July 7, 2010.

6. Temel JS, Greer JA, Muzikansky A, et al. Early palliative care for patients with metastatic non-small-cell lung cancer. N Engl J Med 2010;363(8):733–42.

7. Balduyck B, Hendriks J, Lauwers P, et al. Quality of life evolution after lung cancer surgery: a prospective study in 100 patients. Lung Cancer 2007;56(3): 423–31.

8. Brunelli A, Socci L, Refai M, et al. Quality of life before and after major lung resection for lung cancer: a prospective follow-up analysis. Ann Thorac Surg 2007;84(2):410–6.

9. Paull DE, Thomas ML, Meade GE, et al. Determinants of quality of life in patients following pulmonary resection for lung cancer. Am J Surg 2006;192(5):565–71.

10. Balduyck B, Hendriks J, Lauwers P, et al. Quality of life evolution after lung cancer surgery in septuagenarians: a prospective study. Eur J Cardiothorac Surg 2009;35(6):1070–5.

11. Handy JR Jr, Child AI, Grunkemeier GL, et al. Hospital readmission after pulmonary resection: prevalence, patterns, and predisposing characteristics. Ann Thorac Surg 2001;72(6):1855–9 [discussion: 1859–60].

12. Leo F, Scanagatta P, Vannucci F, et al. Impaired quality of life after pneumonectomy: who is at risk? J Thorac Cardiovasc Surg 2010;139(1):49–52.

13. Sarna L, Padilla G, Holmes C, et al. Quality of life of long-term survivors of non-small-cell lung cancer. J Clin Oncol 2002;20(13):2920–9.

14. Cykert S, Kissling G, Hansen CJ. Patient preferences regarding possible outcomes of lung resection: what outcomes should preoperative evaluations target? Chest 2000;117(6):1551–9.

15. Rocco G, Vaughan R. Outcome of lung surgery: what patients don't like. Chest 2000;117(6):1531–2.

16. Cooley ME. Symptoms in adults with lung cancer. A systematic research review. J Pain Symptom Manage 2000;19(2):137–53.

17. Evangelista LS, Sarna L, Brecht ML, et al. Health perceptions and risk behaviors of lung cancer survivors. Heart Lung 2003;32(2):131–9.

18. Gotoda Y, Kambara N, Sakai T, et al. The morbidity, time course and predictive factors for persistent post-thoracotomy pain. Eur J Pain 2001;5(1):89–96.

19. Wilkie D, Berry D, Cain K, et al. Effects of coaching patients with lung cancer to report cancer pain. West J Nurs Res 2010;32(1):23–46.

20. Pluijms WA, Steegers MA, Verhagen AF, et al. Chronic post-thoracotomy pain: a retrospective study. Acta Anaesthesiol Scand 2006;50(7):804–8.

21. Perkins FM, Kehlet H. Chronic pain as an outcome of surgery. A review of predictive factors. Anesthesiology 2000;93(4):1123–33.

22. Rogers ML, Duffy JP. Surgical aspects of chronic post-thoracotomy pain. Eur J Cardiothorac Surg 2000;18(6):711–6.

23. Schulte T, Schniewind B, Dohrmann P, et al. The extent of lung parenchyma resection significantly impacts long-term quality of life in patients with non-small cell lung cancer. Chest 2009;135(2):322–9.

24. Chernecky C, Sarna L, Waller JL, et al. Assessing coughing and wheezing in lung cancer: a pilot study. Oncol Nurs Forum 2004;31(6):1095–101.

25. Smith EL, Hann DM, Ahles TA, et al. Dyspnea, anxiety, body consciousness, and quality of life in patients with lung cancer. J Pain Symptom Manage 2001;21(4): 323–9.

26. Dales RE, Belanger R, Shamji FM, et al. Quality-of-life following thoracotomy for lung cancer. J Clin Epidemiol 1994;47(12):1443–9.

27. Sarna L, Cooley ME, Brown JK, et al. Symptom severity 1 to 4 months after thoracotomy for lung cancer. Am J Crit Care 2008;17(5):455–67.
28. Sarna L, Evangelista L, Tashkin D, et al. Impact of respiratory symptoms and pulmonary function on quality of life of long-term survivors of non-small cell lung cancer. Chest 2004;125(2):439–45.
29. Claessens MT, Lynn J, Zhong Z, et al. Dying with lung cancer or chronic obstructive pulmonary disease: insights from SUPPORT. Study to understand prognoses and preferences for outcomes and risks of treatments. J Am Geriatr Soc 2000;48(Suppl 5):S146–53.
30. Hopwood P, Stephens RJ. Depression in patients with lung cancer: prevalence and risk factors derived from quality-of-life data. J Clin Oncol 2000;18(4): 893–903.
31. Uchitomi Y, Mikami I, Kugaya A, et al. Depression after successful treatment for nonsmall cell lung carcinoma. Cancer 2000;89(5):1172–9.
32. Faller H, Bulzebruck H. Coping and survival in lung cancer: a 10-year follow-up. Am J Psychiatry 2002;159(12):2105–7.
33. Maliski SL, Sarna L, Evangelista L, et al. The aftermath of lung cancer: balancing the good and bad. Cancer Nurs 2003;26(3):237–44.
34. Hann D, Baker F, Denniston M, et al. The influence of social support on depressive symptoms in cancer patients: age and gender differences. J Psychosom Res 2002;52(5):279–83.
35. Kuo TT, Ma FC. Symptom distresses and coping strategies in patients with non-small cell lung cancer. Cancer Nurs 2002;25(4):309–17.
36. Walker MS, Zona DM, Fisher EB. Depressive symptoms after lung cancer surgery: their relation to coping style and social support. Psychooncology 2006;15(8):684–93.
37. Hill KM, Amir Z, Muers MF, et al. Do newly diagnosed lung cancer patients feel their concerns are being met? Eur J Cancer Care 2003;12(1):35–45.
38. Downe-Wamboldt B, Butler L, Coulter L. The relationship between meaning of illness, social support, coping strategies, and quality of life for lung cancer patients and their family members. Cancer Nurs 2006;29(2):111–9.
39. Meraviglia MG. The effects of spirituality on well-being of people with lung cancer. Oncol Nurs Forum 2004;31(1):89–94.
40. Sarna L, Brown JK, Cooley ME, et al. Quality of life and meaning of illness of women with lung cancer. Oncol Nurs Forum 2005;32(1):E9–19.
41. Kvale PA, Selecky PA, Prakash UB. Palliative care in lung cancer: ACCP evidence-based clinical practice guidelines (2nd edition). Chest 2007; 132(Suppl 3):368S–403S.
42. Jemal A, Thun MJ, Ries LA, et al. Annual report to the nation on the status of cancer, 1975-2005, featuring trends in lung cancer, tobacco use, and tobacco control. J Natl Cancer Inst 2008;100(23):1672–94.
43. Diacon AH, Bolliger CT. Functional evaluation before and after interventional bronchoscopy in patients with malignant central airway obstruction. Monaldi Arch Chest Dis 2001;56(1):67–73.
44. Ernst A, Feller-Kopman D, Becker HD, et al. Central airway obstruction. Am J Respir Crit Care Med 2004;169(12):1278–97.
45. Prakash UB. Bronchoscopy. In: Murray J, Nadel J, editors. Murray and Nadel's textbook of respiratory medicine. Philadelphia: Saunders; 2005. p. 1617–50.
46. Colt HG, Harrell JH. Therapeutic rigid bronchoscopy allows level of care changes in patients with acute respiratory failure from central airways obstruction. Chest 1997;112(1):202–6.

47. Ball JB, Delaney JC, Evans CC, et al. Endoscopic bougie and balloon dilatation of multiple bronchial stenoses: 10 year follow up. Thorax 1991;46(12):933–5.

48. Coulter TD, Mehta AC. The heat is on: impact of endobronchial electrosurgery on the need for Nd-YAG laser photoresection. Chest 2000;118(2):516–21.

49. Schumann C, Hetzel M, Babiak AJ, et al. Endobronchial tumor debulking with a flexible cryoprobe for immediate treatment of malignant stenosis. J Thorac Cardiovasc Surg 2010;139(4):997–1000.

50. Moghissi K, Dixon K, Stringer M, et al. The place of bronchoscopic photodynamic therapy in advanced unresectable lung cancer: experience of 100 cases. Eur J Cardiothorac Surg 1999;15(1):1–6.

51. Wood DE. Airway stenting. Chest Surg Clin N Am 2001;11(4):841–60.

52. Colt HG, Meric B, Dumon JF. Double stents for carcinoma of the esophagus invading the tracheo-bronchial tree. Gastrointest Endosc 1992;38(4):485–9.

53. Freitag L, Tekolf E, Steveling H, et al. Management of malignant esophagotracheal fistulas with airway stenting and double stenting. Chest 1996;110(5): 1155–60.

54. Shin JH, Song HY, Ko GY, et al. Esophagorespiratory fistula: long-term results of palliative treatment with covered expandable metallic stents in 61 patients. Radiology 2004;232(1):252–9.

55. van den Bongard HJ, Boot H, Baas P, et al. The role of parallel stent insertion in patients with esophagorespiratory fistulas. Gastrointest Endosc 2002;55(1): 110–5.

56. Amjadi K, Voduc N, Cruysberghs Y, et al. Impact of interventional bronchoscopy on quality of life in malignant airway obstruction. Respiration 2008;76(4):421–8.

57. Corner J, Hopkinson J, Fitzsimmons D, et al. Is late diagnosis of lung cancer inevitable? Interview study of patients' recollections of symptoms before diagnosis. Thorax 2005;60(4):314–9.

58. Gottlieb LS, Hillberg R. Endobronchial tamponade therapy for intractable hemoptysis. Chest 1975;67(4):482–3.

59. Hiebert CA. Balloon catheter control of life-threatening hemoptysis. Chest 1974; 66(3):308–9.

60. Saw EC, Gottlieb LS, Yokoyama T, et al. Flexible fiberoptic bronchoscopy and endobronchial tamponade in the management of massive hemoptysis. Chest 1976;70(5):589–91.

61. Swersky RB, Chang JB, Wisoff BG, et al. Endobronchial balloon tamponade of hemoptysis in patients with cystic fibrosis. Ann Thorac Surg 1979;27(3): 262–4.

62. Valipour A, Kreuzer A, Koller H, et al. Bronchoscopy-guided topical hemostatic tamponade therapy for the management of life-threatening hemoptysis. Chest 2005;127(6):2113–8.

63. Hetzel MR, Smith SG. Endoscopic palliation of tracheobronchial malignancies. Thorax 1991;46(5):325–33.

64. Morice RC, Ece T, Ece F, et al. Endobronchial argon plasma coagulation for treatment of hemoptysis and neoplastic airway obstruction. Chest 2001; 119(3):781–7.

65. Jain PR, Dedhia HV, Lapp NL, et al. Nd:YAG laser followed by radiation for treatment of malignant airway lesions. Lasers Surg Med 1985;5(1):47–53.

66. Shaw P, Agarwal R. Pleurodesis for malignant pleural effusions. Cochrane Database Syst Rev 2004;1:CD002916.

67. Warren WH, Kalimi R, Khodadadian LM, et al. Management of malignant pleural effusions using the Pleur(x) catheter. Ann Thorac Surg 2008;85(3):1049–55.

68. Putnam JB Jr, Light RW, Rodriguez RM, et al. A randomized comparison of indwelling pleural catheter and doxycycline pleurodesis in the management of malignant pleural effusions. Cancer 1999;86(10):1992–9.

69. Tremblay A, Mason C, Michaud G. Use of tunnelled catheters for malignant pleural effusions in patients fit for pleurodesis. Eur Respir J 2007;30(4):759–62.

70. Olden AM, Holloway R. Treatment of malignant pleural effusion: PleuRx catheter or talc pleurodesis? A cost-effectiveness analysis. J Palliat Med 2010;13(1):59–65.

71. Baker GL, Barnes HJ. Superior vena cava syndrome: etiology, diagnosis, and treatment. Am J Crit Care 1992;1(1):54–64.

72. Rowell NP, Gleeson FV. Steroids, radiotherapy, chemotherapy and stents for superior vena caval obstruction in carcinoma of the bronchus: a systematic review. Clin Oncol (R Coll Radiol) 2002;14(5):338–51.

73. Bierdrager E, Lampmann LE, Lohle PN, et al. Endovascular stenting in neoplastic superior vena cava syndrome prior to chemotherapy or radiotherapy. Neth J Med 2005;63(1):20–3.

74. Chatziioannou A, Alexopoulos T, Mourikis D, et al. Stent therapy for malignant superior vena cava syndrome: should be first line therapy or simple adjunct to radiotherapy. Eur J Radiol 2003;47(3):247–50.

75. Courtheoux P, Alkofer B, Al Refai M, et al. Stent placement in superior vena cava syndrome. Ann Thorac Surg 2003;75(1):158–61.

76. de Gregorio Ariza MA, Gamboa P, Gimeno MJ, et al. Percutaneous treatment of superior vena cava syndrome using metallic stents. Eur Radiol 2003;13(4): 853–62.

77. Garcia Monaco R, Bertoni H, Pallota G, et al. Use of self-expanding vascular endoprostheses in superior vena cava syndrome. Eur J Cardiothorac Surg 2003; 24(2):208–11.

78. Greillier L, Barlesi F, Doddoli C, et al. Vascular stenting for palliation of superior vena cava obstruction in non-small-cell lung cancer patients: a future 'standard' procedure? Respiration 2004;71(2):178–83.

79. Kee ST, Kinoshita L, Razavi MK, et al. Superior vena cava syndrome: treatment with catheter-directed thrombolysis and endovascular stent placement. Radiology 1998;206(1):187–93.

80. Lanciego C, Chacon JL, Julian A, et al. Stenting as first option for endovascular treatment of malignant superior vena cava syndrome. AJR Am J Roentgenol 2001;177(3):585–93.

81. Lau KY, Tan LT, Wong WW, et al. Brachiocephalic-superior vena cava metallic stenting in malignant superior vena cava obstruction. Ann Acad Med Singapore 2003;32(4):461–5.

82. Nicholson AA, Ettles DF, Arnold A, et al. Treatment of malignant superior vena cava obstruction: metal stents or radiation therapy. J Vasc Interv Radiol 1997; 8(5):781–8.

83. Tanigawa N, Sawada S, Mishima K, et al. Clinical outcome of stenting in superior vena cava syndrome associated with malignant tumors. Comparison with conventional treatment. Acta Radiol 1998;39(6):669–74.

84. Urruticoechea A, Mesia R, Dominguez J, et al. Treatment of malignant superior vena cava syndrome by endovascular stent insertion. Experience on 52 patients with lung cancer. Lung Cancer 2004;43(2):209–14.

85. Cepeda MS, Africano JM, Polo R, et al. What decline in pain intensity is meaningful to patients with acute pain? Pain 2003;105(1–2):151–7.

86. Farrar JT, Berlin JA, Strom BL. Clinically important changes in acute pain outcome measures: a validation study. J Pain Symptom Manage 2003;25(5):406–11.

87. Jensen MP. The validity and reliability of pain measures in adults with cancer. J Pain 2003;4(1):2–21.
88. National Comprehensive Cancer Network. Adult pain guidelines 2010. V.1.2010. Available at: www.nccn.org. Accessed August 9, 2010.
89. Paice J. Pain at the end of life. In: Ferrell B, Coyle N, editors. Oxford textbook of palliative nursing. 3rd edition. New York: Oxford University Press; 2010. p. 161–86.
90. Dudgoen D. Dyspnea, death rattle, and cough. In: Ferrell B, Coyle N, editors. Oxford textbook of palliative nursing. 3rd edition. New York: Oxford University Press; 2010. p. 303–20.
91. Jennings AL, Davies AN, Higgins JP, et al. A systematic review of the use of opioids in the management of dyspnoea. Thorax 2002;57(11):939–44.
92. Dudgeon DJ, Lertzman M. Dyspnea in the advanced cancer patient. J Pain Symptom Manage 1998;16(4):212–9.
93. Emtner M, Porszasz J, Burns M, et al. Benefits of supplemental oxygen in exercise training in nonhypoxemic chronic obstructive pulmonary disease patients. Am J Respir Crit Care Med 2003;168(9):1034–42.
94. Vaaler AK, Forrester JM, Lesar M, et al. Obstructive atelectasis in patients with small cell lung cancer. Incidence and response to treatment. Chest 1997;111(1): 115–20.
95. Kvale PA. Chronic cough due to lung tumors: ACCP evidence-based clinical practice guidelines. Chest 2006;129(Suppl 1):147S–53S.
96. Macbeth F, Stephens R. Palliative treatment for advanced non-small cell lung cancer. Hematol Oncol Clin North Am 2004;18(1):115–30.
97. Medley L, Cullen M. Best supportive care versus palliative chemotherapy in nonsmall-cell lung cancer. Curr Opin Oncol 2002;14(4):384–8.
98. Plunkett TA, Chrystal KF, Harper PG. Quality of life and the treatment of advanced lung cancer. Clin Lung Cancer 2003;5(1):28–32.
99. Spiro SG, Rudd RM, Souhami RL, et al. Chemotherapy versus supportive care in advanced non-small cell lung cancer: improved survival without detriment to quality of life. Thorax 2004;59(10):828–36.
100. Thongprasert S, Sanguanmitra P, Juthapan W, et al. Relationship between quality of life and clinical outcomes in advanced non-small cell lung cancer: best supportive care (BSC) versus BSC plus chemotherapy. Lung Cancer 1999;24(1):17–24.
101. Non-Small-Cell Lung Cancer Collaborative Group. Chemotherapy and supportive care versus supportive care alone for advanced non-small cell lung cancer. Cochrane Database Syst Rev 2010;5:CD007309.
102. National Comprehensive Cancer Network. Clinical guidelines in oncology: non-small-cell lung cancer 2010. V.2.2010. Available at: www.nccn.org. Accessed August 9, 2010.
103. Boyar M, Raftopoulos H. Supportive care in lung cancer. Hematol Oncol Clin North Am 2005;19(2):369–87.
104. Borneman T, Koczywas M, Cristea M, et al. An interdisciplinary care approach for integration of palliative care in lung cancer. Clin Lung Cancer 2008;9(6): 352–60.
105. Podnos YD, Borneman TR, Koczywas M, et al. Symptom concerns and resource utilization in patients with lung cancer. J Palliat Med 2007;10(4):899–903.
106. Institute of Medicine. Improving palliative care for cancer. Washington: National Academy Press; 2001.

Palliative Care and Pediatric Surgery

Julia Shelton, MD[a], Gretchen Purcell Jackson, MD, PhD[b],*

KEYWORDS

- Pediatric surgery • Palliative care • Communication
- Ethics • Futility

The American Academy of Pediatrics (AAP) released recommendations regarding pediatric palliative care in 2000.[1] Although the multidisciplinary nature of any pediatric palliative care service was stressed, the role of surgery was not addressed directly, despite pediatric surgeons often being involved in the ongoing treatment of patients with life-limiting conditions. Approximately 400,000 children in the United States are living with a life-threatening disorder. Between 53,000 and 55,000 children die each year,[2] with half dying of chronic, life-long disorders.[3] Many of these children's goals for symptom control at the end of life are not met.[4–7] Pediatric surgeons can play an important role in offering procedures that may improve the quality of life for terminally ill children.

The AAP policy on palliative care states that "the goal is to add life to the child's years, not simply years to the child's life."[1] As more powerful technology allows the physician the means to support and sustain life, the surgeon's role and duty in providing interventions has become controversial, especially in the pediatric population in which there is often a need for the parents to believe that everything possible was done for their child.[3,8] As explained by Mack and Wolfe,[9] "prolonging life, improving symptoms, or maximizing quality of life become appropriate goals when cure is no longer possible." Quality care can only be achieved by having honest discussions about prognosis, developing appropriate treatment goals, and maintaining open lines of communication with patients and their families. Although surgeons may be proficient at discussing the risks and benefits of procedures, they most commonly weigh the risks against long-term benefits, especially in regard to pediatric

This work was supported in part by T32 Research Training Grant No. HS013833 from the Agency for Healthcare Research and Quality.

Financial disclosures/conflicts of interest: the authors have nothing to disclose.

[a] Department of Surgery, Vanderbilt University Medical Center, 1161 21st Avenue South, D-4314 MCN 2730, Nashville, TN 37232-2730, USA

[b] Department of Pediatric Surgery, Vanderbilt Children's Hospital, 2200 Children's Way, 7100 Doctors' Office Tower, Nashville, TN 37232-9780, USA

* Corresponding author.

E-mail address: gretchen.jackson@vanderbilt.edu

patients. In the palliative care setting, these tradeoffs must be put in the context of a shortened life span, and the surgeon must provide realistic expectations for the outcomes of treatment.

This article provides a palliative care primer for the pediatric surgeon. It describes the challenges of providing palliative surgical care in the pediatric population, and provides general guidelines for delivering palliative surgical interventions. Specific pediatric surgical interventions that may be undertaken to achieve palliative goals are also discussed.

CHALLENGES FOR SURGICAL PEDIATRIC PALLIATIVE CARE

Providing surgical palliative interventions in the pediatric population poses unique challenges. Surgical therapies are generally regarded as aggressive treatments, which many do not typically consider as part of a palliative care plan. Because the patients are children, providers and families tend to be more sensitive to the risks of complications, such as postoperative pain, and thus resistant to accepting surgical therapies, even when they have a significant chance of improving overall quality of life. Do-not-resuscitate (DNR) or do-not-intubate (DNI) orders can be obstacles that prohibit the discussion of surgical interventions.

The concept of palliative care is somewhat complicated by the recipients of this care being children, who may not have the intellectual or emotional maturity to understand fully the nature of their condition. The relationship of a surgeon with a pediatric patient must necessarily involve the parents or guardians. Pediatric surgeons are often uniquely rewarded for their work by the patient's potential of a full and productive life.[10] When a child presents with a request for palliative treatment, there exists little hope for a full and productive life. It remains the obligation of the pediatric surgeon to act in the best interest of the patient and to determine, in conjunction with the patient, the family, and other caregivers, what the best interests might be. The trajectory of illness in pediatric patients is often more difficult to predict than in adult patients (**Fig. 1**). This uncertainty can strain an already tenuous relationship between physician, patient, and family.

Families and children involved in the palliative care process are different from their adult counterparts. There often exists a dichotomous goal for parents: the persistent hope for a miracle as new medicines, procedures, or therapies become available; and the pursuit of freedom from pain and unnecessary suffering. It is common for parents to request continued aggressive therapy while insisting that the child be kept as comfortable as possible. Practitioners may have a similar conflict in wanting to extend the boundaries of science and medicine to offer that miracle and wishing to provide the child and their family with a dignified death.

Handling such conflicts can be difficult because both surgeons and pediatricians may have limited training in palliative care. There is no literature that specifically addresses the role of the pediatric surgeon in palliative care. One survey of pediatric surgery residents confirmed that these trainees felt underprepared to confront the moral conflicts that surrounded them in their daily work. They reported significant discomfort in addressing their apprehensions, especially "the pursuit of surgical treatments in 'hopeless' situations, particularly when such treatments resulted in additional complications and suffering for the patients and their families."[11] In another study of pediatricians, Kaneja and Milrod[12] found that few pediatric residents considered themselves equipped to deal with end-of-life issues, and even practicing pediatricians expressed a desire for more support in dealing with death and dying.

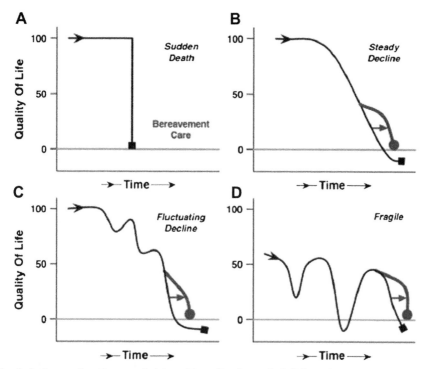

Fig. 1. Patterns of pathways of dying. (*From* Feudtner C. Collaborative communication in pediatric palliative care: a foundation for problem-solving and decision-making. Pediatr Clin North Am 2007;54(5):587; with permission.)

GUIDELINES FOR DELIVERING SURGICAL PALLIATIVE CARE TO CHILDREN

It is critical for pediatric surgeons to have a thorough understanding of the palliative care process to offer interventions in this setting. Palliative care encompasses the concepts of managing "patients with active, progressive, far advanced disease for whom the prognosis is limited and the focus of care is the quality of life."[13,14] It is not a passive process but an active one, and thus, contrary to commonly held beliefs, even surgical interventions may play an important role. Aggressive treatment of symptoms is advocated, including management of pain, anxiety, and gastrointestinal symptoms, whereas actions that do not alter the plan of care (eg, daily laboratory measurements) should be limited.[14] Kon and Ablin[5] submit that palliative care should be referred to as "palliative treatment," and Calabrese[3] recommends the phrase "aggressive care therapy."

Pediatric practitioners may be ideally suited to delivering palliative interventions because they are accustomed to doing procedures in a manner that minimizes anxiety and discomfort, from using local anesthetic before starting intravenous lines to undertaking typical bedside procedures such as chest tubes in the operating room to allow for use of a broad-spectrum analgesic, anesthetic, and amnestic agents. However, this compassionate attitude may discourage pediatric providers from considering surgical therapies in the palliative care setting because of concerns about the risks of anesthesia and postoperative pain. By emphasizing the active nature of palliation, clinicians may be more likely to include operative procedures in their armamentarium, and parents and patients may be more willing to use them. Although potentially perceived as merely semantics, Kon and Ablin[5] as well as Calabrese[3] argue that aggressive palliation is truly a conceptual shift.

Palliative care services for pediatric patients have been steadily increasing in number in the past 2 decades. These dedicated services offer multidisciplinary care for many pediatric patients with life-limiting illnesses, and they address the physical, psychological, and social needs of the patient and family. Pediatric surgeons have historically cared for some of the sickest patients in the hospital, and thus it is reasonable to assume that they would play an important role in a palliative care team. The surgeon's expertise at communicating risks and benefits can be invaluable in discussions regarding the plan of care for patients with life-limiting illness, whether surgical candidates or not.

The general principles for pediatric palliative, end-of-life, and bereavement care include providing appropriate care for an individual patient's care needs, remembering to include both the child and family; ensuring ongoing care from diagnosis through to bereavement; including all providers who may be able to meet the care needs of the patient and family; developing systems necessary to meet these care needs, including education of individuals and organizations; and participating in research to evaluate the current delivery of palliative care and develop improvements.[15]

To achieve the best possible care in the palliative setting, the patient, family, and caregivers must participate in ongoing discussions about the prognosis and goals of care. Multiple investigators suggest that early communication can alleviate strain and facilitate the identification and achievement of goals.[3,14,16–18] The goals for palliative interventions must be clearly defined and updated as the patient's illness progresses. Although there is no strict consensus among all caregivers or parents, most agree that it is reasonable to discuss the child's illness and prognosis to the level of the child's ability to understand.[14,17] It is important to communicate with patients in an age-appropriate manner.[6] Hilden and colleagues[19] confirm that children benefit from discussing their illness as well as their prognosis, and may "feel tremendous isolation if they are not given permission to talk openly about their illness and impending death." However, many parents still ask whether to discuss end-of-life issues with their children. One retrospective study of parents whose children had died of cancer examined whether parents regretted talking with their children about death. Overall, of the parents who had discussed death with their children, none regretted having done so. Although most parents who had not discussed death with their children also did not regret their decision, 27% of parents did regret not speaking about death with their children.[20]

The terms coordinated care or integrated care have been used to describe the dual emphasis on finding a cure for a child's disease and maintaining the comfort of the child throughout the progression of the illness.[1,3] Although these goals may be considered in adults to be incompatible, their coexistence is more often the rule than the exception in pediatric palliative care. Parents do not like doctors to tell them that there is nothing more to be done.[14] They do not want to be perceived as giving up, and, as Calabrese[3] explains, "after their child has died, they must feel that they did everything that could have been done for their child."[3] It is important for health care providers to help the family believe that together they are doing everything for the child to achieve the mutually agreed palliative goals such as relief of symptoms or control of pain.[14]

Surgeons may become involved with the care of terminally ill children in several ways. In some cases, the surgeon may have an established relationship with the patient, perhaps having provided a procedure, such as a tumor resection, earlier in the course of disease when cure was the primary goal. Pediatric surgeons have a uniquely intimate relationship with patients and their families, and, when the treatment goals become palliative, the surgeon may have an important role in helping a family weigh the risks and benefits of additional surgical interventions. Even when operations are not part of the palliative care plan, surgeons can offer their presence, which may provide comfort to the family.

Surgeons are sometimes consulted later in the course of disease with the hope that they can provide a life-saving or life-prolonging procedure on a terminally ill child. The surgeon is considered to be the last hope to regain, if not cure, some sense of normalcy for a period of time. It is, therefore, sometimes left to the surgeon to review the goals of the patient and family and to determine which goals are attainable. The goals of care must be clearly defined when considering surgical interventions. There are times when procedures are not appropriate, either as palliation or in pursuit of a cure. In these situations, it is imperative that all parties involved communicate that the intervention is not consistent with the goals of care. These conversations can be difficult for the surgeon and unbearable for parents who want believe that they are doing everything.

Unreasonable expectations and a lack of clearly defined goals can lead to conflicts among members of the care team, including the patient and family. Although most palliative cases are without conflict regarding end-of-life goals and care,[14,21] the few in which conflict cannot be resolved attract attention because of the ensuing ethical debates regarding patient suffering, quality of life, futility, and resource use. Ethics consultation should be considered to facilitate discussion of these complex issues.[1] Providers cannot be forced to deliver care that they do not think is indicated or beneficial. In some cases, the care of the patient can be transferred to another physician or institution that is willing to provide controversial care. In most situations, ongoing communication of prognosis and emphasis on aggressive management of symptoms to achieve quality of life can aid the patient, family, and health care providers in coming to consensus about realistic goals.

When palliative surgical interventions are consistent with treatment goals, DNR orders may serve as obstacles to patients receiving these procedures. Some surgeons and anesthesiologists insist that such orders be rescinded if patients wish to undergo palliative surgery. Children with terminal illnesses may be more likely than the average patient to have adverse anesthetic reactions and less likely to tolerate the stress of surgery, and, thus, more prone to cardiopulmonary arrest in the operating room or perioperative period. Many practitioners are unwilling to offer procedures that could be considered to hasten the patient's death.[22]

However, terminally ill patients and their families may have legitimate reasons for wanting to maintain DNR orders. If cardiopulmonary arrest occurs, the process of resuscitation may leave the patient in a worse condition than before surgery. In this situation, the operative procedure would likely have failed to achieve the palliative goals, and interoperative death might be viewed by the patient and family as a desirable outcome. Some practitioners advocate honoring preoperative DNR and DNI orders (if the procedure can be done without intubation) during palliative surgery, as long as the patient and the family clearly understand and accept the risks of death.[22] Policies regarding DNR and DNI orders in the perioperative setting vary across institutions and practitioners, and each patient in palliative care has unique wishes and concerns that warrant careful consideration. When palliative procedures are undertaken in patients with DNR or DNI orders, it is the responsibility of the surgeon to address explicitly the increased risks of cardiopulmonary arrest and to discuss the patient's and family's wishes for resuscitation during the perioperative period. Surgeons are not obligated to offer procedures that are certain, or highly likely, to produce arrest, but they should be open to considering the patient's desires should an unintended arrest occur. In this setting, it is important to emphasize that treatments, such as fluid resuscitation or transfusion, can be provided to prevent arrest, and that families have the option of tailoring their DNR orders to permit certain types of resuscitation that they deem acceptable (eg, allowing administration of inotropic agents but not chest compressions).[22]

The situation has been compared with palliation with analgesics or sedatives that can produce significant respiratory depression. In a survey of caregivers providing end-of-life care in the pediatric intensive care unit, most providers agreed that hastening death is an acceptable, unintended side effect of making the patient more comfortable.[23] Clinicians in this study "believe that they were allowing an inexorably moribund patient to die and do not see the cause of death as attributable to the absence of life-support modalities or the provision of sedation and analgesia but rather the underlying disease itself."[23] This double effect, a good act that may be associated with bad consequences, is acceptable in situations in which the intervention is performed to relieve symptoms and not to cause death.

Palliative care is an evolving discipline, and all physicians who participate in palliative care should have opportunities for ongoing education. The AAP recommends that "all general and subspecialty pediatricians, family physicians, pain specialists, and pediatric surgeons need to become familiar and comfortable with the provision of palliative care to children. Residency, fellowship training, and continuing education programs should include topics such as palliative medicine, communication skills, grief and loss, managing prognostic uncertainty, and decisions to forgo life-sustaining medical treatment, spiritual dimensions of life and illness, and alternative medicine."[1] An ethics curriculum has been developed to address the lack of directed ethics training in pediatric surgery. Further research is necessary to determine whether the curriculum is meeting the identified needs.

PALLIATIVE CARE PROCEDURES IN PEDIATRIC SURGERY

Any procedure performed for the benefit of symptom control without treatment of the condition can be deemed palliative. Kon and Albin[5] describe such procedures as palliative therapy, and not as palliative care, to emphasize that treatment is being administered. Even when the goals of treatment become palliative, there remain many things that providers can offer to the patient and the family. However, it should be remembered that there is a great difference between aggressive treatment and unnecessary treatment. The AAP recommends that "for children living with life threatening or terminal conditions, medical professionals are obligated to ensure that medical technology is used only when the benefits for the child outweigh the burdens."[1] Other investigators suggest that "the contemporary test in pediatrics for whether an intervention is ethically appropriate is the best-interest standard – a weighing of expected burdens and benefits of that intervention for a particular child."[24] The indications, risks, and benefits of common pediatric surgical procedures are discussed later.

Gastrostomy

Palliative gastrostomy tube placement is performed to establish enteral access for the administration of medications or nutrition or for venting to relieve or provide comfort from an intestinal blockage. Once such access is established and treatments are administered, issues of withdrawal can arise. Ethical principles dictate that withdrawal of a treatment (eg, stopping enteral feedings) should be considered to be the same as not providing the treatment, but this can be a difficult concept to explain to a family. It may be useful to define parameters regarding when to stop providing medications and nutrition through the tube before the procedure. Although some consider withholding nutrition to be unacceptable, providing nutrition may increase discomfort.[24] Conversely, lack of nutrition may be beneficial at the end of life because it promotes ketosis and endorphin production. Lack of nutrition can decrease symptoms such as nausea, emesis, diarrhea, coughing, and increased respiratory secretions and urine output.[25,26]

Gastrointestinal symptoms such as nausea, vomiting, anorexia, cachexia, constipation, and diarrhea are common among children receiving palliative care. Attention to, and treatment of, these symptoms must be a constant part of any child's palliative care plan. Gastrointestinal symptoms secondary to fasting are also easily addressed.[24] Alternatives to enteral nutrition, such as parenteral nutrition, have not been shown to be beneficial in cachectic or anorexic patients.[27] Some comfort may be provided by tube feedings through a gastrostomy or other temporary feeding tube, but patients and parents should understand that providing enteral feeds cannot reverse the metabolic process of cachexia. Palliative venting gastrostomy has been shown to be effective reducing nausea and vomiting in adult patients with malignant obstruction; its efficacy in children has not been well documented.[28]

Pain Control

Pain control is an important aspect of pediatric palliative care, and although there is literature regarding the management of pain at the end of life, there are few published data on interventional palliative care procedures in children. Medical management of pain according to the World Health Organization 3-step analgesic ladder is a common approach. The addition of adjunct medications for neuropathic pain or atypical methods for pain and anxiety of psychological origin should not be overlooked.[29–32]

It is uncommon for children to experience intense, localized pain amenable to interventional techniques. In these situations, there may be developmental and logistical considerations that complicate the use of interventional techniques in pediatric palliative care; children may not understand the procedures and their role in providing comfort. They may even misunderstand or be unhappy with the results of the treatment (eg, a painful extremity may become completely numb, which may be upsetting to a child or parent). Children also frequently require general anesthesia to undergo such procedures, which may be a substantial risk in this population of patients near the end of life. However, if the risks are clearly understood and the benefits conform with the palliative goals of the patient and the family, then any procedure that potentially offers benefit (eg, an epidural catheter for analgesic delivery) may be worth considering. Case reports have shown image-guided celiac plexus blockade to provide weeks to months of relief from intractable upper abdominal pain in children.[33] Additional research is needed to investigate the efficacy of palliative pain interventions in the pediatric population.

Thoracostomy and Pleurodesis

Chronic pleural effusion is a condition associated with a variety of malignancies that can be seen in pediatric patients at the end of life. There are case reports of the successful treatment of malignant effusions with tube thoracostomy followed by pleurodesis. Of the 7 patients in one case series,[34] all were successfully treated and given the option for discharge to home. Five of the patients elected for discharge; 2 patients elected to continue end-of-life care in the hospital. In weighing the risks and benefits of intervention, patients and parents must be advised that the chest tubes produce pain, and pleurodesis is not always successful in preventing reaccumulation of malignant effusions. The evidence for the efficacy of this procedure is limited, and it is unlikely that the unsuccessful series were submitted for publication.

Tracheostomy

Another common symptom of respiratory distress at the end of life is dyspnea. Medical management is available for both the metabolic and psychological disturbances that may lead to the perception of breathlessness. Noninvasive methods such as supplemental oxygen and positive pressure intermittent ventilation are commonly used. Medications such as opioids and benzodiazepines can also reduce dyspnea. In situations for which these therapies are not sufficient, palliative tracheostomy is an option. This procedure is typically performed for patients who have difficulty swallowing or maintaining their airway, or who experience recurrent aspiration events.[35] For patients with deconditioning or other physiologic decline, tracheostomy may permit the patient to maintain or resume a certain quality of life. Tracheostomy may also permit caregivers to safely transition care for the patient to an outpatient setting.

As with all palliative procedures, it is important to establish specific goals for this intervention. A multidisciplinary approach is recommended, in this case using the services of speech therapists. The disadvantages of tracheostomy must be discussed to ensure that the patient and family understand that speech and swallowing function may be lost. Chan and Devaiah[36] recommend evaluation with 3 questions in considering a tracheostomy: (1) Does the patient understand and desire this intervention and its alternatives? (2) Will this intervention facilitate palliation or supportive care? (3) Do the benefits of the procedure outweigh the risks? These questions are applicable to all decisions about palliative interventions.

Surgical Interventions with Limited Potential for Cure

There are other special situations in which surgical intervention offers a small chance of curative treatment, but more likely serves as the basis for initiating end-of-life care. Laparotomy can be the definitive diagnostic test in certain situations. Once a diagnosis has been established, treatment or palliation can be discussed. For example, in a neonate with gastrointestinal malrotation with midgut volvulus or severe necrotizing enterocolitis, the emergency laparotomy may allow the potential for life-saving treatment or may identify complete bowel ischemia. In the latter situation, the child can be taken to the intensive care unit for discussions with the family. A clear bowel bag can be placed to provide the surgeon with a window to monitor the bowel and the family with the means to understand the child's life-threatening condition.

Surgical resection of lung metastases from osteosarcoma is another example of a procedure that is not considered curative, but may extend life and potentially address symptoms. Resection in these cases is generally considered the standard of care, even for recurrent metastases if complete resection can be achieved without causing respiratory insufficiency and the patient is free of local recurrence or metastases beyond the lung.[37] Resections such as those for desmoid tumors are similarly poised to potentially cure, but are more likely to relieve significant discomfort and allow patients to resume their desired activities.[38] As with all palliative procedures, the risks and benefits of these aggressive interventions must be evaluated in the context of the patient's goals.

SUMMARY

Palliative care is an active process that involves the aggressive management of symptoms to optimize quality of life in terminally ill patients, and operative procedures may have an important role as palliative treatments. As with all palliative interventions, surgical therapies should be evaluated in the context of explicitly defined treatment goals. With pediatric patients, these goals are often defined by parents who need to believe that everything possible was done to help their children. Pediatric surgeons are commonly involved in the care of critically ill children, and it is essential that they become active members in the multidisciplinary team that provides palliative care. The delivery of palliative surgical interventions requires ongoing evaluation of treatment goals and weighing the risks and benefits of procedures in the context of a shortened life span. There is limited published evidence about the efficacy of pediatric palliative procedures, and further research is needed to enable informed discussions of the risks and benefits of interventions in this population.

ACKNOWLEDGMENTS

The authors would like to acknowledge Stephen R. Hays, MD, FAAP for sharing his thoughts about the current use of invasive procedures for pain control in pediatric palliative care.

REFERENCES

1. American Academy of Pediatrics. Committee on Bioethics and Committee on Hospital Care. Palliative care for children. Pediatrics 2000;106(2 Pt 1):351–7.
2. Heron M, Sutton PD, Xu J, et al. Annual summary of vital statistics: 2007. Pediatrics 2010;125(1):4–15.
3. Calabrese CL. ACT–for pediatric palliative care. Pediatr Nurs 2007;33(6):532–4.
4. Heller KS. Integrating palliative and curative approaches in the care of children with life-threatening illnesses: an interview with Ann Goldman 2000. Available at: http://www2.edc.org/lastacts/archives/archivesMarch00/featureinn.asp. Accessed January 10, 2011.
5. Kon AA, Ablin AR. It's not palliative care, it's palliative treatment. Lancet Oncol Feb 2009;10(2):106–7.
6. Himelstein BP, Hilden JM, Boldt AM, et al. Pediatric palliative care. N Engl J Med 2004;350(17):1752–62.
7. Wolfe J, Grier HE, Klar N, et al. Symptoms and suffering at the end of life in children with cancer. N Engl J Med 2000;342(5):326–33.
8. Rushton CH, Hogue EE. When parents demand "everything". Pediatr Nurs 1993;19(2):180–3.
9. Mack JW, Wolfe J. Early integration of pediatric palliative care: for some children, palliative care starts at diagnosis. Curr Opin Pediatr 2006;18(1):10–4.
10. Caniano DA, Ells C. Ethical considerations. In: O'Neill JA, Coran AG, Fonkalsrud EW, et al, editors. Grosfeld: pediatric surgery. 6th edition. Philadelphia (PA): Mosby; 2006. Chapter 14.
11. Chiu PP, Hilliard RI, Azzie G, et al. Experience of moral distress among pediatric surgery trainees. J Pediatr Surg 2008;43(6):986–93.
12. Khaneja S, Milrod B. Educational needs among pediatricians regarding caring for terminally ill children. Arch Pediatr Adolesc Med 1998;152(9):909–14.
13. Meier DE, Morrison RS, Cassel CK. Improving palliative care. Ann Intern Med 1997;127(3):225–30.
14. Masri C, Farrell CA, Lacroix J, et al. Decision making and end-of-life care in critically ill children. J Palliat Care 2000;16(Suppl):S45–52.
15. Field MJ, Behrman RE, editors. When children die: improving palliative and end-of-life care for children and their families. Washington, DC: The National Academies Press; 2003. p. 8–18.

16. Feudtner C. Collaborative communication in pediatric palliative care: a foundation for problem-solving and decision-making. Pediatr Clin North Am 2007;54(5):583–607, ix.
17. Nitschke R, Meyer WH, Sexauer CL, et al. Care of terminally ill children with cancer. Med Pediatr Oncol 2000;34(4):268–70.
18. Himelstein BP. Palliative care for infants, children, adolescents, and their families. J Palliat Med 2006;9(1):163–81.
19. Hilden JM, Watterson J, Chrastek J. Tell the children. J Clin Oncol 2000;18(17):3193–5.
20. Kreicbergs U, Valdimarsdottir U, Onelov E, et al. Talking about death with children who have severe malignant disease. N Engl J Med 2004;351(12):1175–86.
21. Davis JK. Futility, conscientious refusal, and who gets to decide. J Med Philos 2008;33(4):356–73.
22. Walker RM. DNR in the OR. Resuscitation as an operative risk. JAMA 1991;266(17):2407–12.
23. Burns JP, Mitchell C, Outwater KM, et al. End-of-life care in the pediatric intensive care unit after the forgoing of life-sustaining treatment. Crit Care Med 2000;28(8):3060–6.
24. Diekema DS, Botkin JR. Clinical report–forgoing medically provided nutrition and hydration in children. Pediatrics 2009;124(2):813–22.
25. Winter SM. Terminal nutrition: framing the debate for the withdrawal of nutritional support in terminally ill patients. Am J Med 2000;109(9):723–6.
26. Carter BS, Leuthner SR. The ethics of withholding/withdrawing nutrition in the newborn. Semin Perinatol 2003;27(6):480–7.
27. Santucci G, Mack JW. Common gastrointestinal symptoms in pediatric palliative care: nausea, vomiting, constipation, anorexia, cachexia. Pediatr Clin North Am 2007;54(5):673–89, x.
28. Brooksbank MA, Game PA, Ashby MA. Palliative venting gastrostomy in malignant intestinal obstruction. Palliat Med 2002;16(6):520–6.
29. Collins JJ, Grier HE, Kinney HC, et al. Control of severe pain in children with terminal malignancy. J Pediatr 1995;126(4):653–7.
30. Friedrichsdorf SJ, Kang TI. The management of pain in children with life-limiting illnesses. Pediatr Clin North Am 2007;54(5):645–72, x.
31. Collins JJ, Dunkel IJ, Gupta SK, et al. Transdermal fentanyl in children with cancer pain: feasibility, tolerability, and pharmacokinetic correlates. J Pediatr 1999;134(3):319–23.
32. Queinnec MC, Esteve M, Vedrenne J. Positive effect of regional analgesia (RA) in terminal stage paediatric chondrosarcoma: a case report and the review of the literature. Pain 1999;83(2):383–5.
33. Goldschneider KR, Racadio JM, Weidner NJ. Celiac plexus blockade in children using a three-dimensional fluoroscopic reconstruction technique: case reports. Reg Anesth Pain Med 2007;32(6):510–5.
34. Hoffer FA, Hancock ML, Hinds PS, et al. Pleurodesis for effusions in pediatric oncology patients at end of life. Pediatr Radiol 2007;37(3):269–73.
35. Ullrich CK, Mayer OH. Assessment and management of fatigue and dyspnea in pediatric palliative care. Pediatr Clin North Am 2007;54(5):735–56, xi.
36. Chan T, Devaiah AK. Tracheostomy in palliative care. Otolaryngol Clin North Am 2009;42(1):133–41, x.
37. Briccoli A, Rocca M, Salone M, et al. Resection of recurrent pulmonary metastases in patients with osteosarcoma. Cancer 2005;104(8):1721–5.
38. Young-Spint M, Guner YS, Meyers FJ, et al. Radical palliative surgery: new limits to pursue. Pediatr Surg Int 2009;25(10):917–21.

Palliative Care in Urology

Jennifer N. Wu, MD[a], Frederick J. Meyers, MD, MACP[b],
Christopher P. Evans, MD[a],*

KEYWORDS

- Urology - Cancer - Pain - Palliative care

In 2010, genitourinary cancers are expected to account for approximately 29% of the 1.52 million estimated new cancer cases in the United States.[1] Urological malignancies, especially prostate cancer, are relatively common, but patients may live many years before eventually dying of the disease. On the other end of the spectrum, in 25% of patients with newly diagnosed renal cancer, the disease has already metastasized and patients may often die within months of diagnosis. Caring for these patients is an important role for urologists, although medical training often does not adequately prepare urologists for the palliative care of patients with advanced malignancies. In general, the urological community is reluctant to operate for palliation alone when curative intent is not feasible. The usual emphasis on curative therapy leaves many clinicians inexperienced in the various treatment options available for palliative care, including palliative surgery. Furthermore, palliative care is no longer equated with end-of-life care, but rather integrated throughout illness, even when cure is impossible.[2] This rather new concept of simultaneous care, places responsibility on the medical community to offer cancer therapy in concert with supportive care, which includes intensive support of patients and their families. This article focuses on the various palliative treatments available for the 3 most common urological malignancies: prostate, bladder, and renal cancers.

PROSTATE CANCER

Urologists are trained to deal with the morbidity of early prostate cancer therapies, such as impotence and incontinence; however, they are not as well versed in dealing with the symptoms of advanced prostate cancer. Various debilitating symptoms, including bone pain, lymphedema, urinary tract obstruction, and spinal compression, affect patients' quality of life as the disease progresses. Various treatment options are

The authors have nothing to disclose.
a Department of Urology, UC Davis Cancer Center, UC Davis Medical Center, University of California, Davis, 4860 Y Street, Suite 3500, Sacramento, CA 95817, USA
b Department of Internal Medicine, UC Davis Cancer Center, UC Davis School of Medicine, University of California, Davis, 4610 X Street, Suite 3101, Sacramento, CA 95817, USA
* Corresponding author.
E-mail address: cpevans@ucdavis.edu

Surg Clin N Am 91 (2011) 429–444
doi:10.1016/j.suc.2010.12.001
0039-6109/11/$ – see front matter © 2011 Elsevier Inc. All rights reserved.

available to provide comfort and support to patients as these symptoms arise. Androgen deprivation therapy should be the initial treatment of advanced prostate cancer. Impotence, hot flashes, bone loss, and weight gain are side effects of the therapy and should be adequately addressed during treatment. As the cancer progresses, becoming castration resistant, discontinuing the androgen receptor blockade therapy has been shown to temporarily improve symptoms.[3]

Bone Pain

Skeletal metastases are found in 70% of patients with advanced prostate cancer and in more than 90% of patients who die of prostate cancer.[4] The most common locations of metastasis are the pelvis and spine. The sequela of metastases is pain, specifically bone pain in prostate cancer. The achy, burning, or stabbing sensation may be diffuse or localized and may increase at night. Although the exact mechanism of bone pain is unknown, it is likely related to cancer-induced osteolysis. Bone pain not only has an inflammatory and a neuropathic component but also seems to have unique neurochemical features that differ from either component.[5] The treatment options available at present reliably achieve pain control with little toxicity; these options include radiotherapy of bone lesions, decreasing tumor-induced bone loss, surgical stabilization of osteolytic weight-bearing bones, and intensive use of narcotic analgesics (opioids).

Radiation treatment can eradicate bone tumors, thus it can relieve pain caused by tumor burden. About 90% of patients undergoing external beam radiation for palliation of pain experience some pain relief and 54% report a period of complete pain relief. However, the pain in 50% of those patients experiencing partial pain relief will return to pretreatment levels.[6] External beam radiation should be used to treat symptomatic focal metastasis in order to limit tissue damage and minimize anemia. Long bone involvement necessitates treatment of the full length of the bone to prevent tumor recurrence in the marrow and intramedullary sites. Surgical stabilization before radiation treatment is required for weight-bearing bones, with greater than 50% of the cortex seen to be eroded on plain radiograph or computed tomographic scan. Patients with disseminated tumors can be treated with strontium 89, a bone-seeking radioisotope that is administered intravenously.[7,8] Strontium 89 is a calcium analogue, which is deposited by osteoblasts near metastatic tumors. Shallow-penetrating low-energy beta particles are emitted, thus limiting damage to surrounding tissues. Pain may initially increase, but 80% of patients will eventually have reduction in pain with 10% showing complete relief lasting 3 to 6 months.[9] This radioisotope should not be used for urgent conditions, such as spinal cord compression, because several weeks of treatment are required to show benefit. Sufficient bone marrow reserves must be present before treatment. Care must be taken to rule out metastatic masses that may become edematous and compress the spinal cord after treatment. Other possible side effects include anemia, pancytopenia, and pneumonitis. Samarium Sm 153 lexidronam (Sm 153) is a similar radiopharmaceutical that has been shown to be effective in treating bone pain from metastatic prostate cancer.[10,11] This radiopharmaceutical has a chelator moiety that associates with hydroxyapatite crystals that are concentrated in areas of bone turnover, thus delivering beta- and gamma-emitting radioisotopes to areas of osteoblastic bone metastasis. Mild and transient bone marrow suppression has been associated with Sm 153. Repeat dosing of Sm 153 has been shown to be efficacious and well tolerated in patients in whom the bone pain returns after an initial dose.[12]

In contrast to radiation therapy, chemotherapy has not been as effective for the palliation of pain. The Cochrane Database performed a systematic review of randomized trials evaluating different chemotherapeutic regimens for hormone-refractory prostate cancer and concluded that the most promising therapy was that using doce-taxel plus prednisone.[13] A randomized trial compared docetaxel plus prednisone with mitoxantrone plus prednisone, which was the most common chemotherapeutic treat-ment for pain related to hormone-refractory prostate cancer. A total of 35% of patients treated with docetaxel experienced reduction in pain compared with 22% of patients treated with mitoxantrone. Quality of life improved with response rates of 23% and 13%, respectively.[14] A follow-up analysis of the TAX 327 study was recently published confirming that survival of men with metastatic hormone-resistant prostate cancer is significantly longer after treatment with docetaxel and prednisone than with mitoxan-trone and prednisone.[15]

Most bone metastases from prostate cancer are osteoblastic, but significant oste-oclastic activity does occur.[16] Bisphosphonates work by binding to bone surfaces undergoing active remodeling to inhibit osteoclast activity and bone resorption, result-ing in reduction of pain.[17] Early-generation bisphosphonates showed little clinical benefit in prostate cancer but were effective in treating primarily osteolytic lesions from multiple myeloma and breast cancer, whereas the currently used third-generation medications are much more potent.[18] Zoledronic acid (4 mg) was given intravenously over 15 minutes every 3 weeks for 15 months in a prostate cancer trial. At all recorded time points, reported pain scores were lower, with significant reduction at 3 and 9 months. The risk of skeletal-related events, such as fractures, was reduced by 36%, and the onset of the first skeletal-related event was delayed by 321 days.[19] As a result of reducing osteoporosis, bisphosphonates can be useful in asymptomatic patients undergoing androgen deprivation therapy.[20] Recently, 2 new drugs have been shown in separate randomized double-blind placebo-controlled phase 3 clinical trials to reduce the incidence of fractures in men on androgen deprivation therapy. Denosumab, a fully humanized monoclonal antibody against the receptor activator of nuclear factor $\kappa\beta$ ligand, has been shown to increase the bone mineral density and decrease the rate of new vertebral fractures in men receiving androgen depriva-tion therapy for nonmetastatic prostate cancer.[21] Denosumab was recently approved by the Food and Drug Administration (FDA) for the treatment of men with prostate cancer receiving hormone therapy. Use of toremifene, a selective estrogen receptor modulator, also showed a decreased rate of vertebral fractures in patients with pros-tate cancer, 4.9% in the placebo group versus 2.5% in the toremifene group.[22] Tore-mifene is FDA approved for use in metastatic breast cancer and is currently being reviewed for use in men with prostate cancer on hormone therapy. **Fig. 1** is a summary of the treatment options for bone pain.

Glucocorticoids can reduce bone pain, but the mechanism is unclear. The inhibition of prostaglandin release may prevent hypersensitization of peripheral nerves and reduce edema near lesions to decrease pressure. Typically, oral prednisone, 20 to 40 mg/d, is effective, but even lower equivalent doses have been used. Glucocorti-coids should be used as a bridge between more long-acting treatments because pain reduction is usually short lived. Glucocorticoids and nonsteroidal antiinflamma-tory drugs (NSAIDs) should not be used together because toxicity is increased but analgesia is not synergistic.

Although the previously mentioned treatments deal with the cause and pathophys-iology of pain, analgesics can be used to alter how pain is experienced. After a reliable assessment of pain severity is completed for mild pain, treatment should begin with oral acetaminophen or NSAIDs.[23] Opioids are the mainstay for moderate to severe pain and can be combined with NSAIDS or acetaminophen. Once the pain is under control with an initial short-acting morphine, a long-acting form with limited supply of the short-acting form for breakthrough pain is appropriate (**Fig. 2**). Although

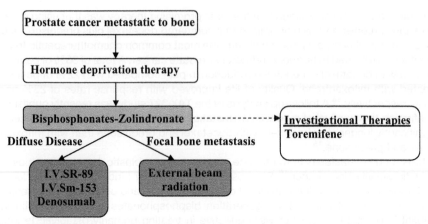

Fig. 1. Simplified treatment algorithm for bone pain secondary to prostate cancer. Darker gray in boxes denotes increasing treatment aggressiveness. IV, intravenous; Sm 153, Samarium 153; Sr 89, strontium 89. (*From* Ok JH, Meyers FJ, Evans CP. Medical and surgical palliative care of patients with urological malignancies. J Urol 2005;174:1177; with permission.)

overdosage is rarely a problem, undertreatment of pain is a frequent quality-of-care issue. Dosages can be increased until adequate pain relief is achieved or until adverse effects become intolerable. There is no maximum dosage for most opioids, but opioids that contain acetaminophen should not exceed the maximum daily dose of 3500 mg/d and considerably less in elderly patients and patients with known liver disease. Stool softeners and stimulant laxatives should be added to the regimen as patients will likely to have opioid-induced constipation. Often, an escalating regimen of stimulant laxatives and enemas may be required for severe constipation. Most importantly, the clinician should attempt to make an accurate assessment and then reassessment of the pain severity before, during, and after intervention. This consensus-validated approach to pain management is shown in **Fig. 2.**

Pelvic Pain

Prostate cancer with local advancement into the rectum and sacral plexus can cause severe perineal pain. After conventional treatments, such as hormone deprivation or

Mild to moderate pain — NSAIDs, acetaminophen, acetylsalicylic acid.	Equianalgesic dose po. (mg)	
	Morphine	30
	Hydrocodone	30
Moderate pain Opioids : codeine, dihydrocodeine, oxycodone, hydrocodone	Hydromorphone	7.5
	Levorphonal	1
	Methadone	2.4
Severe pain Opioids : morphine, hydromorphone, methadone, fentanyl, Levorphanol	Oxycodone	20
	Codeine	200

Fig. 2. Analgesics for bone pain. Medication options for different intensities of pain and narcotic dosage conversions for common medications are shown. (*From* Ok JH, Meyers FJ, Evans CP. Medical and surgical palliative care of patients with urological malignancies. J Urol 2005;174:1177; with permission.)

radiation therapy, fail and when systemic analgesia is not adequate or has an unacceptable side effect profile to systemic analgesics, regional analgesia procedure performed by an anesthesia pain expert should be considered. In patients with well-preserved functional performance status, surgeons may consider total pelvic exenteration in highly selected cases. A small retrospective study of patients with locally recurrent prostate cancer showed that all patients had significant pain reduction. Furthermore, 79% of patients had complete pain relief with a mean symptom-free period of 14.1 months.[24] **Fig. 3** shows the progressive treatments for pelvic pain.

Bladder Outlet Obstruction

During any stage of prostate cancer, men may experience urinary tract obstruction. Enlarging tumors can compress the prostatic urethra, invade the bladder, or obstruct a ureteral orifice. Besides bothersome voiding symptoms, bladder outlet obstruction can result in urine accumulation in the bladder, causing lower abdominal pain and pressure. If left untreated, hydronephrosis and renal failure may ensue. An indwelling urinary catheter or a percutaneous suprapubic catheter is required during episodes of acute obstruction. Evaluation for azotemia and retention before the use of nephrotoxic medications is required for all patients.

For patients not on androgen deprivation therapy, hormone manipulation is often effective in reducing bladder obstruction. Within 3 to 6 weeks after hormone levels reach castrate levels, patients may be able to void. Transurethral resection of the prostate (TURP) is an option if hormonal therapy fails. Crain and colleagues[25] reported their retrospective series of patients with advanced prostate cancer undergoing palliative TURP and showed that patients had significant improvement in urinary symptoms. The International Prostate Symptom Score improved from 21.1 preoperatively to 11.0 postoperatively. However, patients undergoing a palliative TURP had higher postoperative urinary retention and reoperation rates when compared with patients undergoing a TURP for benign prostatic hyperplasia. Often, repeat resection may be required to remove additional obstructing tissue, but it may also be done to control local bleeding. Postresection hematuria can be controlled with continuous irrigation, and mild traction of an inflated urethral catheter for up to 24 hours may be helpful. In a select group of patients with bladder invasion from prostate cancer, cystoprostatectomy can be effective for palliation of obstructive symptoms and reduce the need for drainage catheters.[26] Urethral stents are an option for obstruction if a patient cannot tolerate a transurethral resection procedure or refuses long-term catheter placement. Although stent placement is successful in 88% to 100% of patients, it should only be offered to patients with a limited life expectancy. Tumor growth into

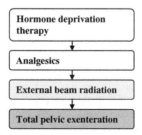

Fig. 3. Simplified treatment algorithm for pelvic pain in prostate cancer. (*From* Ok JH, Meyers FJ, Evans CP. Medical and surgical palliative care of patients with urological malignancies. J Urol 2005;174:1177; with permission.)

the stent is common and will eventually cause obstruction. Radiation therapy is another effective treatment for reducing obstruction.

Ureteral Obstruction

Hydronephrosis, azotemia, and renal failure are avoidable results of untreated tumor extension into the bladder trigone or compression of the ureter/ureterovesical junction by enlarging retroperitoneal lymph nodes causing obstruction.[27,28] These are common results of locally extensive tumors involving the seminal vesicles and the periprostatic tissue surrounding the bladder. More than 50% of patients have bilateral ureteral obstruction.

Radiation therapy is effective for these patients, with 70% response rates in previously untreated patients.[29] A faster working treatment is hormonal therapy, which can result in an 85% response rate.[30] Retrograde placement of ureteral stents via cystoscopy is often difficult in patients with significant obstruction. Alternatively, percutaneous nephrostomy tubes can be placed easily and provide immediate relief of obstruction. If the patient desires an internal ureteral stent, it can be placed antegrade through the nephrostomy site. Urologists should be aware that exchanging stents cystoscopically may be difficult, especially if tumor has invaded the distal ureter and trigone. The treatment options for obstruction are summarized in **Fig. 4**.

Spinal Cord Compression

Among patients with castration-resistant prostate cancer, 10% have spinal cord compression. The possible causes of compression are vertebral collapse from tumor invasion or pressure from extradural growth along the spinal cord. The most common locations of cord compression are the thoracic and upper lumbar spine.[31] All patients experience severe pain, often radicular in distribution, with other possible symptoms including sensory deficits, lower extremity motor weakness, and hypotonic neurogenic bladder. Although progression of symptoms may be slow, rapid onset of paraplegia (within 24–36 hours) or bladder dysfunction is a sign of spinal cord vascular insufficiency and poor recovery of function. Surgical intervention may be the patient's best option to reduce permanent neurologic damage. Plain radiographs or bone scans are used to confirm the approximate location of compression, after it is identified by neurologic examination. However, magnetic resonance imaging provides the best detail of the spinal cord and surrounding structures. Outcome is related to the neurologic status before treatment, but the overall treatment response is greater than 50%.

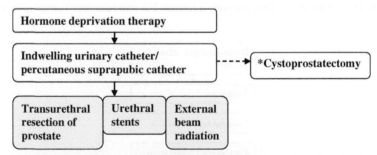

Fig. 4. Simplified treatment algorithm for ureteral and bladder outlet obstructions in prostate cancer. The asterisk indicates that cystoprostatectomy is considered for select patients. (*From* Ok JH, Meyers FJ, Evans CP. Medical and surgical palliative care of patients with urological malignancies. J Urol 2005;174:1177; with permission.)

Performance status and extent of disease elsewhere should be considered when considering operative intervention. Immediately upon diagnosis, edema surrounding the spinal cord must be reduced with steroids.[32,33] Usually, dexamethasone, 100 mg, is given intravenously followed by 16 to 64 mg/d. Although the standard treatment of spinal cord compression caused by metastatic cancer is corticosteroids and radiotherapy, Patchell and colleagues[34] published a randomized trial showing that direct decompressive surgery plus postoperative radiotherapy is superior to radiotherapy alone. Both groups in this trial received initial steroid therapy upon diagnosis. Although the patients in this study had mixed primary tumor histologic findings, 30% of tumors were of genitourinary origin. Patients treated with surgery retained the ability to walk significantly longer than those with radiotherapy alone (median 122 days vs 13 days). The surgical approach and procedure depends on tumor location and severity of spinal damage.[35] Radiation therapy alone for spinal compression is an option.[36] Areas of previous radiotherapy with compression may need surgical decompression. Most patients who are able to ambulate before surgery usually retain the ability after treatment; however, only 50% of patients regain the ability.[37] **Fig. 5** shows the 2 treatment pathways for slow and rapid progression of spinal cord compression.

BLADDER CANCER

Urothelial carcinoma (UC), formerly called transitional cell carcinoma, is the most common bladder cancer in the United States and Europe. Metastatic UC is aggressive, with a median survival of less than 1 year. This condition is associated with debilitating symptoms of bleeding, pain, dysuria, and urinary obstruction. Typically, noninvasive treatments, such as intravesical therapy and radiation therapy, are attempted initially. If these treatments fail, invasive options are available, which include laser vaporization, laser resection, transurethral resection, arterial embolization, urinary diversion alone, and palliative cystectomy with urinary diversion. Treatment of urinary obstruction has already been discussed in the section on prostate cancer.

Bleeding/Pain

Patients with advanced cancer having bleeding should initially be screened for a coagulopathy. If clot evacuation and ϵ-aminocaproic acid (Amicar) treatment fail to control

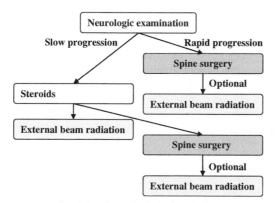

Fig. 5. Simplified treatment algorithm for spinal cord compression in prostate cancer. (*From* Ok JH, Meyers FJ, Evans CP. Medical and surgical palliative care of patients with urological malignancies. J Urol 2005;174:1177; with permission.)

the bleeding, several intravesical treatments are available. Bladder irrigation with 1% to 2% alum (potassium or ammonium aluminum sulfate) or 1% silver nitrate can be effective.[38] If renal insufficiency is present or bladder lesions allow a significant amount of alum to enter the vascular system, serum aluminum levels should be monitored. Patients can typically tolerate these intravesical treatments, so anesthesia is not usually required.

Formalin instillation is effective in controlling hematuria but carries a greater risk, including perforation and bladder fibrosis.[39] Formalin, at 2.5% to 4% concentration, is instilled passively until half the bladder capacity is reached and left inside for 20 to 30 minutes. Then the bladder is irrigated continuously with normal saline. Because this procedure is painful, general or regional anesthesia is required. Reflux should first be ruled out with an intraoperative cystogram. If reflux is present, balloon catheters should be inserted into the lower part of the ureters and the patient placed in reverse Trendelenburg position to prevent formalin reflux and subsequent upper tract damage.[40]

Another treatment option includes radiation therapy, which is commonly used to control bleeding and pain. In one study, up to 59% of patients with advanced bladder cancer had resolution of hematuria and 73% had pain reduction after treatment.[41] In another study, complete palliation of locally advanced bladder cancer was found in 43% of patients.[42] Although bladder and bowel complications are possible, radiation therapy is generally well tolerated. Chemotherapy has not been as well studied for palliation of pain or bleeding in advanced bladder cancer. Possible chemotherapeutic agents for palliation include cisplatinum and methotrexate, but they are not as effective as radiation.

Laser resection or vaporization is a viable minimally invasive alternative for both superficial and invasive lesions. A more invasive treatment option is transurethral resection, which may control symptoms more effectively. After conservative methods have failed, embolization or surgical ligation of hypogastric arteries may be required. Cystectomy with urinary diversion should only be considered in patients with good performance status if all other options have failed or are not feasible because it is the most invasive treatment associated with the greatest morbidity. The various treatments for bleeding and pain are depicted in **Fig. 6**.

RENAL CELL CARCINOMA

At presentation, 20% to 30% of patients with renal cell carcinoma (RCC) will have metastatic disease and less then 30% of patients treated for localized RCC will progress to have metastatic disease.[43] Nonlocalized RCC is aggressive with a 5-year survival rate of less than 10%.[44] However, the use of vascular endothelial growth factor inhibitors or tyrosine kinase inhibitors have extended the life expectancy from 12 months to as high as 24 months. Regardless, palliation remains an essential goal in metastatic RCC because it is resistant to radiation and chemotherapy. Several effective palliative options are available to treat the paraneoplastic syndromes, local tumor progression, bleeding, pain, and respiratory compromise that can be associated with advanced RCC.

Paraneoplastic Syndrome

Occasionally, patients with RCC have paraneoplastic syndromes. The most common paraneoplastic syndrome associated with RCC is cancer anorexia-cachexia syndrome (CACS), defined as anorexia, involuntary weight loss, tissue wasting, poor performance, and ultimately, death. CACS should be suspected if a patient has

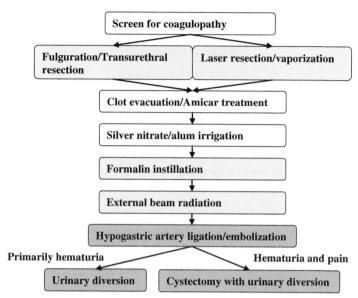

Fig. 6. Simplified treatment algorithm for bleeding/pain caused by bladder cancer. All the treatment steps are not required. Some treatments will be bypassed depending on the severity of the symptoms. (*From* Ok JH, Meyers FJ, Evans CP. Medical and surgical palliative care of patients with urological malignancies. J Urol 2005;174:1177; with permission.)

involuntary weight loss of more than 5% of preillness weight over a 2- to 6-month period. RCC can result in the production of inflammatory cytokines, which can manifest as fever, night sweats, anorexia, weight loss, protein catabolism, and dysgeusia (the altered sensation of taste resulting in food tasting and smelling bad). Treatment regimen of either a low-dose corticosteroid, hydrocortisone, 20 mg twice a day, or progesterone, 800 mg/d, is equally effective. However, responses are often transient. Other manifestations include hypercalcemia from parathyroid hormone–related peptide, erythrocytosis from erythropoietin production, hypertension from renin, and nonmetastatic hepatic dysfunction from granulocyte-macrophage colony-stimulating factor. If symptoms continue after nephrectomy, metastatic disease is present and prognosis is poor.

Bleeding/Pain

Although radiation therapy provides no survival advantage, it can reduce the size of symptomatic tumors and possibly facilitate resection of left-sided tumors. Because of possible damage to the liver, right-sided tumors are typically not treated with radiation. Infarction of tumor by arterial embolization is another treatment option with possible side effects including renal failure and damage to nontarget organs. However, this treatment option is effective for controlling bleeding, pain, and hypertension.[45] An epidural catheter placed before embolization can decrease postprocedure narcotic requirements and ileus related to postembolization syndrome. An algorithm of treatments for RCC is shown in **Fig. 7**.

Up to 40% of patients with metastatic RCC develop osseous metastasis.[46] Treatments for palliation of bone pain are similar to those of prostate cancer, with the exception of hormone therapy. Additional therapy includes selective transcatheter embolization of painful RCC skeletal metastases.[47] However, it should be noted

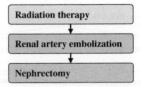

Fig. 7. Simplified treatment algorithm for bleeding/pain caused by RCC. (*From* Ok JH, Meyers FJ, Evans CP. Medical and surgical palliative care of patients with urological malignancies. J Urol 2005;174:1177; with permission.)

that when this therapy is used for vertebral metastases paralysis is a major potential complication.

Palliative Surgery

Palliative nephrectomy for locally advanced and metastatic RCC is the most aggressive treatment option.[48] Palliative nephrectomy differs from cytoreductive surgery; the latter has been shown to improve survival in patients undergoing immunotherapy and is currently under investigation for use with tyrosine kinase inhibitors. Palliative nephrectomy can be performed to prevent future hematuria, anemia, or pain, and it can ameliorate some paraneoplastic symptoms.[49] However, careful patient selection is required because of the significant morbidity associated with the surgery. There is also a psychological aspect of removing the primary tumor that may play a role in the decision to undergo nephrectomy.[50] Approximately 4% to 10% of patients with RCC have a tumor thrombus in the inferior vena cava (IVC) and 1% have tumor thrombus into the atrium.[51] Patients with these conditions in the face of metastatic disease may decide to undergo a nephrectomy with IVC/atrial thrombectomy because it may improve quality of life and prolong survival by ameliorating a potential pulmonary embolus.[52] Aggressive surgery can also possibly relieve symptoms of pain and other burdensome symptoms. **Figs. 8** and **9** demonstrate the operative approach to maximize exposure for a right-sided cytoreductive radical nephrectomy with IVC thrombectomy. Ligation of the short hepatic veins and rotation of the liver to the left upper quadrant facilitate infrahepatic vena caval occlusion and thrombectomy.

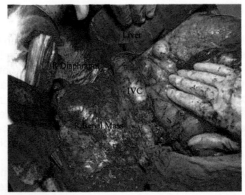

Fig. 8. Intraoperative photograph of cytoreductive right radical nephrectomy for stage T3c tumor. R diaphragm, right side of diaphragm; R renal mass, right renal mass.

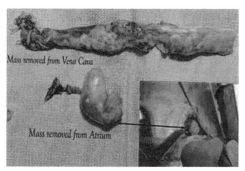

Mass removed from Vena Cava

Mass removed from Atrium

Fig. 9. Photograph of the thrombus removed from vena cava and atria during cytoreductive nephrectomy.

Endobronchial Obstruction and Bleeding

Metastatic tumors of the lung are relatively rare but can obstruct airways and cause bleeding. If lesions are central, laser phototherapy is successful in reducing both obstruction and bleeding. The effectiveness decreases with peripheral lesions, increasing degree of obstruction, and length of obstruction.[53]

SIMULTANEOUS INVESTIGATIONAL THERAPY AND SUPPORTIVE CARE

The World Health Organization defines palliative care as "an approach that improves the quality of life of patients and their families facing the problem associated with life-threatening illness, through the prevention and relief of suffering by means of early identification and impeccable assessment and treatment of pain and other problems, physical, psychosocial and spiritual."[54] The primary goal of palliative care is to reduce suffering.

When proven curative therapies have failed, patients may wish to participate in clinical trials. The concept of simultaneous care allows patients to be involved in clinical trial and receive palliative care. A study performed at the authors' institution showed that simultaneous administration of investigational and palliative care can be provided without adverse events.[2,55] More patients in the simultaneous care group than in the usual care group opted for hospice care. Psychometric variability among patients likely accounted for the lack of statistical significance in evaluating quality-of-life measures. A randomized controlled study, project Educate, Nurture, Advise, Before Life Ends (ENABLE), showed that patients receiving telephone-based psychoeducational intervention have an improved quality of life and mood compared with patients receiving usual oncologic care only.[56] Of the 322 participants in the study, 12% had cancer of the genitourinary tract. A more recent nonblinded randomized controlled trial conducted at the Massachusetts General Hospital compared quality of life and mood in patients with metastatic non–small cell lung cancer receiving standard oncologic care alone with that in patients receiving standard oncologic care with palliative care.[57] Using the Functional Assessment of Cancer Therapy-Lung scale and the Hospital Anxiety and Depression Scale, researchers found that patients receiving standard oncologic care with palliative care had better quality of life and fewer depressive symptoms than patients receiving standard oncologic care alone. In addition, the palliative care group received less aggressive end-of-life care and had a longer median survival of 2.7 months ($P = .02$). Although this cohort of patients was specific to metastatic non–small cell lung cancer, the results are promising for all patients with metastatic disease dealing with end-of-life issues. The investigators proposed that with earlier referral to hospice programs, patients would receive care with better management of symptoms, leading to stabilization of their condition and prolonged survival, although this hypothesis will require further studies. However, Medicare regulatory barriers prevent simultaneous hospice care and disease-directed therapy payments in both the prehospice and posthospice phases. Medicare coverage for hospice services is available for 2 periods of 90 days and an unlimited number of 60-day periods.[58] Regarding hospitalized patients in whom terminal care and death is imminent (whether from cancer, vascular disease, chronic infection, or other diseases), primary physicians should seek palliative care consultation when available. Approximately 40% of hospitals in California offer this service. It is also important to use the V code for these patients, which is appropriate and beneficial for billing and improves the mortality index of the hospital in several hospital-ranking formulas.

Although simultaneous care is still evolving, it may be a useful tool in the treatment of urological malignancies, especially metastatic RCC. As mentioned earlier in this article, metastatic RCC is difficult to treat because chemotherapy and radiation therapy are not effective. For a select group of patients interested in clinical trials, nephrectomy may be necessary because certain experimental treatments require pathologic examination of the nephrectomy specimen for enrollment. Some tumor vaccine strategies require sizeable pathologic specimens in order to purify tumor-infiltrating lymphocytes or tumor tissue.[59,60] After nephrectomy, some patients may even experience a postoperative improvement in performance status, possibly increasing tolerance of subsequent systemic therapy. There are also ongoing clinical trials, such as the Adjuvant Sorafenib or Sunitinib in Unfavorable Renal Cell Carcinoma (ASSURE) trial, evaluating the use of adjuvant cytokine therapy in patients with metastatic RCC after undergoing a nephrectomy.

Curative therapy and palliative care should not be viewed as separate entities in which one excludes the other. Instead of curative therapy ending when palliative care begins, there should be a smooth transition from mostly curative therapy to mostly palliative care.[61] If patients choose to continue aggressive experimental therapy, there should still be a transition to include palliative care. It is appropriate to consider palliative aspects of care at the time of diagnosis of any serious or life-limiting illness.

SUMMARY

Patient suffering begins at the initial diagnosis of cancer because there is a tremendous amount of stress caused by an uncertain future, the prospect of death, leaving behind loved ones, and fear of physician abandonment. Over time, most patients with newly diagnosed cancer adapt to the crisis of the diagnosis and the subsequent treatments, but there is a wide range in the coping ability.[62] At certain points along disease progression, such as metastasis to bone, the additional stress may be overwhelming and supplemental professional or family support may be needed. Physicians should anticipate these events and aid in preparing patients and their support network in order to minimize suffering. One difficult task of physicians is estimating the patient's survival and determining an appropriate timeline for enrollment in hospice care. Medicare hospice benefits require documentation by a primary care physician and hospice medical director that a patient's expected prognosis does not exceed 180 days when enrolled in hospice care.[58] A recent study from the Urologic Diseases of America Project analyzed the Surveillance, Epidemiology and End Results-Medicare database and found that just more than 50% of patients who died of prostate cancer used hospice care.[63] Although this study showed an increased rate of hospice enrollment over the past decade, the timing of enrollment remains poor.

Enrollment within 7 days of death was noted in 22% of hospice users, whereas 9% of hospice users enrolled more than 180 days before death. This study showed the benefits of hospice care because patients enrolled in hospice care were less likely to receive high-intensity care, including intensive care unit admissions, inpatient stays, and multiple emergency department visits. Hospice care can be beneficial, but hospice stays shorter than 7 days are too brief to maximize the benefit of enrollment. The investigators propose the appropriate timing of hospice care enrollment to be between 7 and 180 days before death.

Physicians should have an ongoing conversation with patients about personal goals, prognosis, uncertainty of outcome, reassurance of continued physician involvement, and discussion of the resources available, especially enrollment into hospice programs. Palliative care should be a standard part of every urology practice because urologists will be dealing with oncologic malignancies throughout their career.

REFERENCES

1. Jemal A, Siegel R, Xu J, et al. Cancer statistics, 2010. CA Cancer J Clin 2010; 60(5):277–300.
2. Meyers FJ, Linder J. Simultaneous care: disease treatment and palliative care throughout illness. J Clin Oncol 2003;21:1412.
3. Scher HI, Zhang ZF, Nanus D, et al. Hormone and antihormone withdrawal: implications for the management of androgen-independent prostate cancer. Urology 1996;47:61.
4. Coleman RE. Skeletal complications of malignancy. Cancer 1997;80:1588.
5. Honore P, Rogers SD, Schwei MJ, et al. Murine models of inflammatory, neuropathic and cancer pain each generates a unique set of neurochemical changes in the spinal cord and sensory neurons. Neuroscience 2000;98:585.
6. Tong D, Gillick L, Hendrickson FR. The palliation of symptomatic osseous metastases: final results of the study by the Radiation Therapy Oncology Group. Cancer 1982;50:893.
7. Brundage MD, Crook JM, Lukka H. Use of strontium-89 in endocrine-refractory prostate cancer metastatic to bone. Provincial Genitourinary Cancer Disease Site Group. Cancer Prev Control 1998;2:79.
8. Patel BR, Flowers WM Jr. Systemic radionuclide therapy with strontium chloride Sr 89 for painful skeletal metastases in prostate and breast cancer. South Med J 1997;90:506.
9. Robinson RG, Preston DF, Schiefelbein M, et al. Strontium 89 therapy for the palliation of pain due to osseous metastases. JAMA 1995;274:420.
10. Sartor O, Reid RH, Hoskin PJ, et al. Samarium-153-Lexidronam complex for treatment of painful bone metastases in hormone-refractory prostate cancer. Urology 2004;63:940.
11. Serafini AN, Houston SJ, Resche I, et al. Palliation of pain associated with metastatic bone cancer using samarium-153 lexidronam: a double-blind placebo-controlled clinical trial. J Clin Oncol 1998;16:1574.
12. Sartor O, Reid RH, Bushnell DL, et al. Safety and efficacy of repeat administration of samarium Sm-153 lexidronam to patients with metastatic bone pain. Cancer 2007;109:637.
13. Mike S, Harrison C, Coles B, et al. Chemotherapy for hormone-refractory prostate cancer. Cochrane Database Syst Rev 2006;4:CD005247.
14. Tannock IF, de Wit R, Berry WR, et al. Docetaxel plus prednisone or mitoxantrone plus prednisone for advanced prostate cancer. N Engl J Med 2004;351:1502.

15. Berthold DR, Pond GR, Soban F, et al. Docetaxel plus prednisone or mitoxantrone plus prednisone for advanced prostate cancer: updated survival in the TAX 327 study. J Clin Oncol 2008;26:242.

16. Lipton A, Small E, Saad F, et al. The new bisphosphonate, Zometa (zoledronic acid), decreases skeletal complications in both osteolytic and osteoblastic lesions: a comparison to pamidronate. Cancer Invest 2002;20(Suppl 2):45.

17. Rodan GA, Reszka AA. Bisphosphonate mechanism of action. Curr Mol Med 2002;2:571.

18. Green JR, Muller K, Jaeggi KA. Preclinical pharmacology of CGP 42'446, a new, potent, heterocyclic bisphosphonate compound. J Bone Miner Res 1994;9:745.

19. Saad F, Gleason DM, Murray R, et al. A randomized, placebo-controlled trial of zoledronic acid in patients with hormone-refractory metastatic prostate carcinoma. J Natl Cancer Inst 2002;94:1458.

20. Smith MR, Eastham J, Gleason DM, et al. Randomized controlled trial of zoledronic acid to prevent bone loss in men receiving androgen deprivation therapy for nonmetastatic prostate cancer. J Urol 2003;169:2008.

21. Smith MR, Egerdie B, Hernandez Toriz N, et al. Denosumab in men receiving androgen-deprivation therapy for prostate cancer. N Engl J Med 2009;361:745.

22. Smith MR, Morton RA, Barnette KG, et al. Toremifene to reduce fracture risk in men receiving androgen deprivation therapy for prostate cancer. J Urol 2010; 184(4):1316–21.

23. Practice guidelines for cancer pain management. A report by the American Society of Anesthesiologists Task Force on Pain Management, Cancer Pain Section. Anesthesiology 1996;84:1243.

24. Kamat AM, Huang SF, Bermejo CE, et al. Total pelvic exenteration: effective palliation of perineal pain in patients with locally recurrent prostate cancer. J Urol 2003;170:1868.

25. Crain DS, Amling CL, Kane CJ. Palliative transurethral prostate resection for bladder outlet obstruction in patients with locally advanced prostate cancer. J Urol 2004;171:668.

26. Leibovici D, Kamat AM, Pettaway CA, et al. Cystoprostatectomy for effective palliation of symptomatic bladder invasion by prostate cancer. J Urol 2005;174:2186.

27. Saitoh H, Yoshida K, Uchijima Y, et al. Two different lymph node metastatic patterns of a prostatic cancer. Cancer 1990;65:1843.

28. Surya BV, Provet JA. Manifestations of advanced prostate cancer: prognosis and treatment. J Urol 1989;142:921.

29. Megalli MR, Gursel EO, Demirag H, et al. External radiotherapy in ureteral obstruction secondary to locally invasive prostatic cancer. Urology 1974;3:562.

30. Michigan S, Catalona WJ. Ureteral obstruction from prostatic carcinoma: response to endocrine and radiation therapy. J Urol 1977;118:733.

31. Rosenthal MA, Rosen D, Raghavan D, et al. Spinal cord compression in prostate cancer. A 10-year experience. Br J Urol 1992;69:530.

32. Grossman SA, Lossignol D. Diagnosis and treatment of epidural metastases. Oncology (Williston Park) 1990;4:47.

33. Loblaw DA, Laperriere NJ. Emergency treatment of malignant extradural spinal cord compression: an evidence-based guideline. J Clin Oncol 1998;16:1613.

34. Patchell RA, Tibbs PA, Regine WF, et al. Direct decompressive surgical resection in the treatment of spinal cord compression caused by metastatic cancer: a randomised trial. Lancet 2005;366:643.

35. Welch WC, Jacobs GB. Surgery for metastatic spinal disease. J Neurooncol 1995;23:163.

36. Smith EM, Hampel N, Ruff RL, et al. Spinal cord compression secondary to prostate carcinoma: treatment and prognosis. J Urol 1993;149:330.

37. Huddart RA, Rajan B, Law M, et al. Spinal cord compression in prostate cancer: treatment outcome and prognostic factors. Radiother Oncol 1997;44:229.

38. Goel AK, Rao MS, Bhagwat AG, et al. Intravesical irrigation with alum for the control of massive bladder hemorrhage. J Urol 1985;133:956.

39. Donahue LA, Frank IN. Intravesical formalin for hemorrhagic cystitis: analysis of therapy. J Urol 1989;141:809.

40. Sarnak MJ, Long J, King AJ. Intravesicular formaldehyde instillation and renal complications. Clin Nephrol 1999;51:122.

41. Srinivasan V, Brown CH, Turner AG. A comparison of two radiotherapy regimens for the treatment of symptoms from advanced bladder cancer. Clin Oncol (R Coll Radiol) 1994;6:11.

42. Salminen E. Unconventional fractionation for palliative radiotherapy of urinary bladder cancer. A retrospective review of 94 patients. Acta Oncol 1992;31:449.

43. Janzen NK, Kim HL, Figlin RA, et al. Surveillance after radical or partial nephrectomy for localized renal cell carcinoma and management of recurrent disease. Urol Clin North Am 2003;30:843.

44. Motzer RJ, Bander NH, Nanus DM. Renal-cell carcinoma. N Engl J Med 1996; 335:865.

45. Kalman D, Varenhorst E. The role of arterial embolization in renal cell carcinoma. Scand J Urol Nephrol 1999;33:162.

46. Swanson DA, Orovan WL, Johnson DE, et al. Osseous metastases secondary to renal cell carcinoma. Urology 1981;18:556.

47. Forauer AR, Kent E, Cwikiel W, et al. Selective palliative transcatheter embolization of bony metastases from renal cell carcinoma. Acta Oncol 2007;46: 1012.

48. Wood CG. The role of cytoreductive nephrectomy in the management of metastatic renal cell carcinoma. Urol Clin North Am 2003;30:581.

49. Mosharafa A, Koch M, Shalhav A, et al. Nephrectomy for metastatic renal cell carcinoma: Indiana University experience. Urology 2003;62:636.

50. Mickisch GH, Mattes RH. Combination of surgery and immunotherapy in metastatic renal cell carcinoma. World J Urol 2005;23:191.

51. Marshall FF, Dietrick DD, Baumgartner WA, et al. Surgical management of renal cell carcinoma with intracaval neoplastic extension above the hepatic veins. J Urol 1988;139:1166.

52. Kirkali Z, Van Poppel H. A critical analysis of surgery for kidney cancer with vena cava invasion. Eur Urol 2007;52:658.

53. Chan AL, Yoneda KY, Allen RP, et al. Advances in the management of endobronchial lung malignancies. Curr Opin Pulm Med 2003;9:301.

54. World Health Organization. Cancer pain relief and palliative care: report of a WHO expert committee (Technical Report Series 804). Geneva (Switzerland): WHO; 1990. p. 11.

55. Meyers FJ, Linder J, Beckett L, et al. Simultaneous care: a model approach to the perceived conflict between investigational therapy and palliative care. J Pain Symptom Manage 2004;28:548.

56. Bakitas M, Lyons KD, Hegel MT, et al. Effects of a palliative care intervention on clinical outcomes in patients with advanced cancer: the Project ENABLE II randomized controlled trial. JAMA 2009;302:741.

57. Temel JS, Greer JA, Muzikansky A, et al. Early palliative care for patients with metastatic non-small-cell lung cancer. N Engl J Med 2010;363:733.

58. Christakis NA, Escarce JJ. Survival of Medicare patients after enrollment in hospice programs. N Engl J Med 1996;335:172.
59. Figlin RA, Thompson JA, Bukowski RM, et al. Multicenter, randomized, phase III trial of CD8(+) tumor-infiltrating lymphocytes in combination with recombinant interleukin-2 in metastatic renal cell carcinoma. J Clin Oncol 1999;17:2521.
60. Jocham D, Richter A, Hoffmann L, et al. Adjuvant autologous renal tumour cell vaccine and risk of tumour progression in patients with renal-cell carcinoma after radical nephrectomy: phase III, randomised controlled trial. Lancet 2004;363:594.
61. Ok JH, Meyers FJ, Evans CP. Medical and surgical palliative care of patients with urological malignancies. J Urol 2005;174:1177.
62. Weisman AD, Worden JW. The existential plight in cancer: significance of the first 100 days. Int J Psychiatry Med 1976;7:1.
63. Bergman J, Saigal CS, Lorenz KA, et al. Hospice use and high-intensity care in men dying of prostate cancer. Arch Intern Med 2010. [Epub ahead of print].

Surgical Palliative Care in Haiti

Joan L. Huffman, MD, CWS

KEYWORDS

• Palliative care • Mass casualty event • Haiti earthquake
• Wound care

13. *We are on our scabbed backs.*
There is the sound of whispered splashing,
And then this:
Leave them.

Patricia Smith

According to the World Health Organization, palliative care is an approach that improves the quality of life of patients and their families facing life-threatening illness through the prevention, assessment, and treatment of pain and other physical, psychosocial, and spiritual problems.[1]

The US Homeland Security definition of a catastrophic health event or mass casualty event (MCE) is "any natural or manmade incident, including terrorism, that results in a number of ill or injured persons sufficient to overwhelm the capabilities of immediate local and regional emergency and healthcare systems."[2] In summary, disaster care at its inception is a minimally acceptable care because of the diversity and volume of patients. In today's world, responders must deal not only with an austere environment with challenges to resources, access, and transport but also with physical, economic, and social difficulties made more complex by political constraints.[3]

What happens when an MCE collides with palliative care? Hurricane Katrina of 2005 is a national example. In 2010, a disaster of even greater magnitude occurred in Haiti, a Pan-American nation located just 600 miles from Florida.

BACKGROUND

Palliative care was initially instituted for better pain control in patients with cancer. As time progressed, it expanded to include symptom control and enveloped not only the physical person but also the emotional and spiritual being. Palliative care now focuses

The author has nothing to disclose.
Division of Acute Care Surgery, Department of Surgery, University of Florida at Shands Jacksonville, 655 West 8th Street, 8th Floor Clinical Center, Jacksonville, FL 32209, USA
E-mail address: joan.huffman@jax.ufl.edu

on the relief of suffering, health care needs, dignity of the person, and quality of life at the end of life. It encompasses the patient's family and friends. Over the past 30 years, additional focus has been placed on the care of patients with AIDS. With the aging of the baby boomers of the North American and European populations, patients with chronic disease states (such as chronic obstructive pulmonary disease, renal failure, and decompensated coronary artery disease/congestive heart failure) are also considered now for palliative care.

What happens to palliative care when an MCE occurs? Following an MCE, there are 4 groups of patients who fall into the "not expected to survive" category: patients already under hospice/palliative care; vulnerable patients in long-term care facilities with an advanced disease (1%–2% of normal population); individuals exposed to the MCE who are expected to die; and other patients triaged due to scarce resources. Suddenly, because of an abruptly austere environment, all these patients are shifted to palliative care.

New Orleans, Louisiana, was overwhelmed with the onslaught of Hurricane Katrina. Despite the high-tech modern health care system of the United States, difficult decisions had to be made in harrowing circumstances. With generator failures, critical care equipment ceased to function, and with modern just-in-time stores and cutoff of supply lines, severe shortages of medication, food, and potable water occurred; both patients and staff suffered immensely. In these circumstances, palliative care was often the best and/or the only care that medical staff could provide. In St. Rita's Nursing Home, St. Bernard Parish, 20 miles southeast of New Orleans, staff abandoned patients whom they could not evacuate. Patricia Smith, a poet, gives voice to each of the 34 individuals who died. Particularly poignant is 13, a resident who was lucid enough to realize that they were being left to drown (see opening quote).[4]

In recognition of the events that happened post-Katrina, a recent ruling by The Joint Commission instructed that "the needs of those who may not survive catastrophic MCE and the 'existing' vulnerable populations affected by the event should be incorporated in to the planning, preparation, response and recovery management systems of all regions and jurisdictions." In addition, surge capacity should be addressed with attention to triage and rationing of supplies and personnel. A defined minimum of what is palliative care, to be made available to all, must take priority over heroic efforts toward severely injured or critically ill patients.[5] Aggressive steps have been taken to implement these recommendations in the United States; other nations are not as fortunate.

HAITI

How does palliative care play out in even more austere circumstances? An opportunity to learn the answer arose on January 12, 2010, when a 7.0 Richter scale earthquake struck Haiti, the poorest country in the Western Hemisphere, and absolute devastation occurred. There were more than 200,000 fatalities, 300,000 injuries, and millions of displaced persons. It was a disaster of epic proportions, and even now in retrospect, one of the major TIME stories of 2010.[6,7]

HISTORICAL PERSPECTIVE

Haitian response to the disaster and subsequent interaction with and expectations of international health care providers must be viewed based on a historical/sociocultural context, health beliefs, and the access to care. Until 1492, and contact by Christopher Columbus, the island was inhabited by indigenous peoples (Taíno/Arawak) who perished after enslavement by the Spanish. They were replaced first by the Nicaraguan slaves and soon after by Africans through the Atlantic slave trade. Eventually, competition between Spanish and French interests led to the division of Hispaniola into a French western one-third and a Spanish eastern two-thirds, the modern day Haiti and Dominican Republic (DR), respectively. Haiti proved profitable to France as its richest colony for over 2 centuries.

In 1804, Haiti became the first Black republic after the slaves fought and won their independence from their colonial masters. Haiti thrived for the following century until external (exploitation by foreign investors and governments) and internal forces (political corruption, instability, and mismanagement) led to the decay of freedom, underdevelopment, and generalized suffering. Only after the end of the Duvalier dictatorship in 1986 and the subsequent 1991 coup d'état of Jean-Bertrand Aristide (by the Toton Macoute, with US collaboration), which ended in 1994, did the most basic of infrastructures evolve under the leadership of President René Préval. This fragile system collapsed, both structurally and functionally, with the earthquake.[8]

SOCIOCULTURAL ASPECTS

Haiti is populated by more than 9 million young individuals: 50% are younger than 20 years, and about half are rural and single. Almost everyone speaks *Kreyòl* (Haitian Creole), a mélange of French, African, Arawakan, Spanish, and English; however, literacy, defined as the ability to read French, is very low (rural, 20%; urban, 50%). The literacy rate is not surprising because three-quarters of the population have just a primary school education. More than 90% of all formal educational institutions are nonstate private facilities; university education is attained by only 1%.

Class hierarchy is powerful, with special focus on economic background, culture, language, and education. Hailing back to colonization, further stratification is based on skin tone. Light-skinned literate persons with access to private education maintain an elite status with most of the social, economic, and political powers, whereas dark-skinned people tend to be marginalized.[8]

The disparity is echoed in income inequality, which is one of the highest worldwide. A small elite of several thousand people includes many millionaires contrasted with the teeming slums of the capital city, Port-au-Prince (P-a-P), where the daily income may be $2. The disparity also resonates in unemployment (one-third of rural persons, one-half of metropolitan dwellers) and basic services (most rural homes have no indoor plumbing, only 10% have electricity compared with 90% with power access in metro regions). In 2008, the gross national income per capita was $653.70; more than 80% of the population lives in poverty, and 54% in abject poverty. Because of the desperate conditions, many Haitians have migrated to the United States (500,000) and Canada (Montreal, 100,000). The annual remittances of the diaspora provide $800 million of support to friends and family in the homeland. The current US recession has drastically reduced remittances at a time of financial desperation in Haiti.[9,10]

An extended, elastic family unit is the basic support structure, with interdependence on clusters of units sharing a common *lakou* (courtyard). In more-urban nonshanty town areas, a combination of time-honored and Anglo elements existed; however, much of these elements have reverted to traditional arrangements with the explosive evolution of tent-city communities.

Fathers, often absent, hold family authority and financial responsibility, but in reality, the mothers are the *poto mitan* (central pillar) of the family. The most common family structure is *viv avek* (living with) common-law unions and their respective 5 to 7 children. Another pattern is *plasaj*, in which a man has more than 1 common-law wife. The man is supposed to provide for each of his wives and the children of their relationship. Legal/religious marriages are encouraged by the state and church for filial and social stability and AIDS prevention. The roles of men reside in financial provision, home maintenance, and agriculture, whereas women run the household and manage the meager budget.

At the extremes of age, elders are treated with high respect in intergenerational households, with the oldest man in the home having authority. On the other hand, children are raised with great discipline and corporal punishment. It is not uncommon for poor rural families, with hopes of better lives for their children, to give their children to foster families. Unfortunately, many of the restavèk (stay with) youths are subject to the abuses of human trafficking.[8]

HEALTH BELIEFS

Health practices in Haiti cannot be discussed in isolation from religion and culture. Haiti has a rich religious diversity that blends Vodou (unknown percentage), Catholic (80%), and Protestant (20%) beliefs. Despite public affiliation with Christianity, most Haitians practice Vodou (the Fon word for spirit) to some degree. After Vodou was forbidden and Catholicism made mandatory, slaves gave their African gods the names of Catholic saints; this naming gave them the superficial appearance of compliance, but they were able to keep facets of their native beliefs. Other African deities are known as lwas (ancestors' spirits) and are considered guardian angels, but they may also "possess" the body of an individual, more commonly women than men. This possession can be confused with mental illness or neurologic disorders. More rural and poorer people perform Vodou rituals, but in times of crisis, even upper-class Haitians may resort to traditional faith for aid. In general, Haitians do not speak openly about Vodou.

In juxtaposition to North American/Western anthropocentric culture, that is, humans are the center of the Universe, Haitians exist in a cosmocentric culture, that is, humans are just 1 form of energy, condensed and drawn from an all-encompassing cosmic Being. The primary focus of this great Being is to bring one into harmony and synergy with the energy of the universe. The concept of the individual is that one is made up of 4 dimensions: kò kadav (body), lonbraj (shade), gwo bon-anj (big good angel), and nam/ti bon-anj (little good angel). In concert with these tenets is a hybrid model of illness and health. There should be a balance between health, the state of well-being in connectedness to nature, the nonhuman environment, family and friends, the human environment, and the invisible, the spirits, and illness, the state of being ill with or disharmony between elements of the environment. Keeping these concepts in mind, illness is thought to originate from the failure to observe rules of hygiene, ethical rules, and rules that govern how humans relate with nature. In the humoral theory, disease is caused by an imbalance of these components. Appropriate treatment is to restore equilibrium by applying treatment in the opposite direction.

Other influences are failure to observe ancestor rites and evil influence of others (human or otherwise).

Illness is classified into 3 domains: maladi Bondyè (God's disease/natural causes), treatment is by either Western medicine or doktè fey (traditional healers); maladi fè-moun mal (human magic spells); and maladi lwa or Satan (good or evil spirits), healing is by consultation with the bòkò (magician) or oungan (Vodou priest, using herbal and ritual practices, or pursuing "unnatural" causes of illness). Oungans are not adverse to biomedical treatments and may refer clients who are beyond their scope of practice. Bòkòs are professional sorcerers who can cast or undo curses/spells or, on the positive side, aid in the achievement of personal gains. Spiritual leaders, both traditional and religious, can be used as allies to encourage patients to follow medical treatments and/or to help obtain trust by serving as cotherapists. Supernatural forces are considered to be the cause of mental illness. The problem is thought to be because of a hex, curse, or failure to please the spirits of the deceased. Death is considered to be just a normal phase of the energy flow through the cycle of life, from birth to life to death to ancestor spirit.

Illness is experienced and described much differently than in Western medicine. Symptoms may be related as metaphors depending on the volatility of the circumstances, with no reference to anatomy but to energy or other natural/unnatural elements. The practitioner is expected to elicit the appropriate symptoms to make a diagnosis.[8]

PREEARTHQUAKE ACCESS TO HEALTH CARE

The Haitian Ministère de la Santé Publique et de la Population budget for health care is $2 per person per year. About 46% of the country's medical professionals work in P-a-P, although 70% of the population lives outside P-a-P. There is high infant mortality, and the average life span of a Haitian is 61 years, with only 3.4% aged more than 65 years compared with 13% in the United States.[11,12]

There is little to no access to health care in rural areas. In the mountain village, where we provided a free clinic for 2 days on our last Haiti mission, the priest, Pere Desca, told us that his community had not seen a doctor for more than a year (Pere Desca, Fond Baptiste, Haiti, personal communication, August 2010). Sadly, more than 80% of trained doctors leave Haiti within 5 years of graduation.

Hôpital de l'Université d'État d'Haiti (HUEH) was the main clinical referral and the only 24-hour trauma center in Haiti. HUEH, known to the people of P-a-P as Hopital General, operated on an annual budget of $5 million. Hopital General, downtown near the National Palace, as well as the national medical school and nursing schools were decimated by the earthquake. An entire class of nursing students was killed. Many hospital staff were killed or injured or had to leave to care for their injured family members.

IMMEDIATE POSTEARTHQUAKE RESPONSE BY HAITIANS

Some of the most vulnerable individuals, the residents of the collapsed Hospice Municipal, a nursing home in Delmas-2 located only a mile from the airport, were left with only the administrator and cleaner to care for them. Of the 94 residents, 6 survived the event and were left lying in the open, some on mattresses and others in the dirt, with rats picking at their overflowing diapers. A carton of water had been donated; 1 family member came with a small amount of boiled rice. Neighboring, Place de la Paix, slum people thronged to the nursing home grounds to set up tents, threatening and stealing their meager belongings. Two elderly people tried to guard the group: a blind man in a wheelchair and an old lady who brandished her walking stick. Day by day, the residents died or waited to die because of dehydration, hunger, and no medicine.[13]

Zanmi Lasante (ZL), the flagship project of Partners in Health (PIH), provided care to the multitudes that fled to Haiti's Central Plateau and Artibonite regions, set up health outposts at 4 camps for internally displaced people in P-a-P, and began working at Hopital General with the 370 remaining staff and volunteers. ZL also facilitated the placement of volunteer surgeons, physicians, and staff, as well as helped the hospital's Haitian leadership.[14]

Max Delices, the director at Hospice St Joseph (HSJ), our team's base camp, told us that before we came, he helped pull people from rubble and mobilized young volunteers to go out into the neighborhood with povidone-iodine (Betadine) and gauze to clean and dress wounds. "Everyone was a doctor in those first hours and days." He said that our visit gave hope for a future to him, the staff, and the neighborhood and that he slept for the first time in more than a week (Max Delices, HSJ, P-a-P, Haiti, personal communication, January 2010).

EARLY RELIEF MISSION RESPONSE

Nearly 1000 members of the American College of Surgeons responded to the disaster. Some of the earliest surgical help arrived from Miami on January 13th, and triage began under tents at the United Nations compound just outside P-a-P. Initial care included intravenous (IV) hydration, morphine analgesia, and oral antibiotics. Amputations were done under local anesthesia. Tetanus toxoid arrived 24 hours later, and the team began to operate in conjunction with an Israeli team. Over the next week, a Civil War camp of tents, additional supplies, and specialists evolved.[15]

The principle of justice was used as disaster teams focused on potentially survivable yet severely injured earthquake survivors. A Haitian facility agreed to provide palliative care to individuals who were under coma, in vegetative states, or minimally responsive or whose families opted for comfort care only. Staff of this facility were trained on the US Naval Ship (USNS) COMFORT for 3 days; supplies were also provided.[16]

A. Brent Eastman, MD, FACS, responded to a hospital 1 mile from the earthquake epicenter, where he scrubbed under a broken faucet and operated on a patient with upper extremity compartment syndrome, with no electric cautery, ketamine-only anesthesia, and no monitoring. The patient's arm was saved, and the patient was satisfied with the care provided. The American team learned the necessity of sensitivity to working in another culture and quickly learned to invite the Haitian technicians to scrub with them and to give the Haitian doctors first choice of operating "rooms" and anesthesiologists. Dr Eastman said, "We were there to help, not to dominate and occupy."[17]

Other important lessons learned were the necessity of reliance on basic physical diagnostic skills, with no laboratories, radiographs, or computed tomographic scans. The doctors had "to look at the patient, talk to the patient and touch the patient," said Sylvia Campbell, MD, FACS. In such dire circumstances, it was a pleasure for physicians and a comfort to patients to participate in the laying on of hands.

A surgical resident, Joseph Sakran, MD, learned the lesson of his young career as he watched a teenage patient with late-stage tetanus and horrific spasmodic contractions. The only care available was supportive. The patient was moved to a dark, quiet room, both for his comfort as he lay dying and to take him out of the tent where his situation had terrified the other patients.[15]

The severity, complexity, and number of survivors taxed the limits of the USNS COMFORT, which arrived within 8 days of the disaster. In a staff meeting, colleagues discussed the difficult decisions confronting them, such as ventilator capacity, blood product use, the conflict between routine trauma management and disaster management, and the allotment of scarce resources. One option included setting up palliative care facilities at triage sites onshore, but a surgeon nixed the idea because he was aghast at the concept of having a tent of dying patients adjacent to a medevac site, and he found it unpalatable to give a bed to a moribund patient. However, nursing argued that a bed out of the sun and painkillers were more humane than leaving the individual to "die in the street under the sun like a dog." During the brief meeting, 2 patients died, 1 in the operating room.[16]

Two doctors, in the Fundamental Disaster Management (FDM) subcommittee of the Society of Critical Care Medicine (SCCM), described their situations on arriving at P-a-P. One was Dennis Amundson, DO, FCCM, who led an 18-member intensivist team of respiratory therapists and nurses as the initial staff on the USNS COMFORT. They cared for critically ill patients in a 40-bed intensive care unit (ICU) at full capacity for 3 weeks. They had to make difficult triage decisions, focusing their attention on patients who "weren't necessarily the sickest, but had the best opportunity for long term survival." Other patients were kept as comfortable as possible until their demise.

The other doctor, James Geiling, MD, FCCM, and 8 nurses from Dartmouth Medical Center teamed up with PIH at Hopital General to set up a postoperative/ICU tent adjacent to an improvised operating room in one of the remaining single- or double-story buildings; all multistory buildings had collapsed, "it looked like it had been bombed."[18] Their team provided critical care to crush and gunshot wound survivors with only a small supply of antibiotics, an oxygen tank, and a blood pressure cuff (until the cuff was stolen). Dr Geiling said, "My ICU management was how strong was their pulse, how pale was their tongue and how fast they were breathing." It was ICU care in name only; in fact, it was wound care and physical diagnosis.[19] As more assistance arrived, teams from the United States and around the world pooled and collaborated. Medical providers worked around the clock in the first hours and days, with more than half of the team members requiring IV hydration; after a few days, operations were cut back to daylight hours only to allow conservation of provider energy because it quickly became obvious that the number was not going to decrease anytime in the foreseeable future.[18]

The earthquake occurred while the 39th Critical Care Congress, SCCM, was in session in Miami, Florida; at that very time, discussions were underway to initiate Fundamental Critical Care Support (FCCS) training in the DR. How ironic because Haiti was not the only country affected by the earthquake disaster, as survivors rushed to the DR, where 75% of the 7.5 million residents use the public hospital system. An SCCM Disaster Field Team (DFT) was quickly formed, and it did an initial assessment of the overflowing Jimani, DR, clinic at the Haiti-DR border and the 70 public ICU beds in the entire DR, which were staffed with nurses with minimal critical care education, had no respiratory therapists, and had minimal equipment. In 3 days, the DFT set up and subsequently taught the earthquake disaster portions of both FDM and Pediatric FCCS to 60 medical residents and nurses, who immediately went to work at the Jimani clinic; 3 weeks later, a repeat course educated another 30 staff members, and a new 6-bed ICU was set up in Barahona, DR. The health systems of both countries of Hispaniola will remain stressed for an extended period.[20]

A team from Operation Smile provided palliative care for a 4-year-old child with more than 85% flame burns, who was not able to access care until postinjury day 3. The best care they could provide was to remove the child's burnt clothing in the operating room, with only morphine for analgesia and silver sulfadiazine (Silvadene) and soft gauze to cover the wounds. The USNS COMFORT was unable to provide burn care, and there were no other burn facilities available. The child's mother was gently told the bad news, and the child was kept as comfortable as possible until his immediate demise.[21]

PERSONAL EXPERIENCE

I had the opportunity to respond to the earthquake disaster 1 week after the event. Our host was the HSJ, not a hospice in American terms but a guesthouse for visiting health care providers and a refuge for people from the countryside, who came to P-a-P seeking medical care. In addition, there was a maternal-infant clinic on-site, and educational scholarships were administered.[22] The building and its surrounding walls had pancaked down as so many did in the few fatal seconds; however, there were no injuries on-site, although one of the directors rode the building down. The staff secured the premises with corrugated aluminum barriers and salvaged mattresses and cooking implements from the rubble. Due to limited space within the confines of our walls, we multi purposed the area: during the day, we held an on-site clinic, at night the same location served as our living room, dining room and bedroom. We slept on the ground with the staff and shared a meal of beans and rice each evening.

Our base was in the Christ Roi neighborhood, a "Red Zone" and a poor area that the government did not prioritize for care. The Disaster Medical Assistance Team (DMAT), shown on the international news, was at the Hopital General in downtown P-a-P and in other "Green Zones" such as Pètionville. Our 13-member team consisted of a surgeon; a family practice intern; a trauma psychologist; a medical nurse practitioner; 2 physician assistants, 1 medical and the other surgical; 2 registered nurses; a social worker; a public health specialist; an anthropologist; and 2 unarmed security men. Among them, 5 members were fluent in Kreyòl. We partnered with 12 local paramedical volunteers to treat people with little to no access to health care in the local neighborhood, the Acra district tent city several blocks away, and the huge Solino tent city set up on a soccer field in one of the city's slum areas.

Our 20 crates of medical supplies were either lost or subverted, so we were limited to the contents of 13 duffel bags that we hand-carried on the chartered flight from Miami. Our supplies consisted of basic wound/fracture care materials, IV/oral rehydration solutions, and basic adult and pediatric medications. These minimal resources were expanded with some additional pediatric drugs salvaged from the HSJ clinic and donated by the Catholic Relief Services and the International Medical Corps.

In 5 days, we treated more than 1000 people from our seemingly bottomless duffel bags; it was truly an example of what can be done with a few supplies and a lot of imagination, a modern day feeding of the multitudes with 7 loaves and 7 fishes. A small contingent of the team held daily clinics at HSJ, but the remainder worked in Klinik Mobil (mobile clinics) in the tent cities. We enlisted local men to construct temporary shaded or screened patient areas; doors balanced on chairs served as examination tables.

We did not see any actively dying people, but the mangled arm of a motorcyclist protruded from the debris in the street. Near Hopital General, body after body was carried into an overflowing morgue. Women crouched curbside, cooking with charcoal, while human excrement ran by their feet; the overpowering sweet stench of death permeated the air, intermingled with the acrid smoke of burning bodies and garbage.

Of the disease categories, 50% were surgical and 50% medical. Every person we examined had lost either a family member or a friend; some had lost all. Many had witnessed the deaths, the tragedy just an arm's length away, yet unreachable. We dealt with the after effects, both physical and emotional. No matter what the presenting problem was, everyone complained of tet fe mal, vant doule, and verti (headache, stomach pain, and dizziness). The source of their ailments was not only acute injury but also ongoing austere conditions, dehydration, hunger, and enormous stress. Neither the patients nor their accompanying person was turned away empty-handed, everyone was given a packet of over-the-counter pain relief and antacids as a simple palliative measure.

Five patients required transport by private vehicle to Hopital General: a man with severe head injury, who was carried into the Klinik with seizures and a distended tender abdomen; a woman with cauda equina syndrome; a man with a lumbar fracture, who was brought on a blanket into the *Klinik* (I made him a thoracolumbar brace from a cardboard box and 2 Ace bandages); and 2 infants with refractory dehydration.

We did not have the capability to provide any extensive operative interventions, except for wound debridement and digital amputations. All surgical procedures were done under local or regional anesthesia, supplemented by oral ibuprofen and emotional support by the team's psychologist or social worker. One young girl passed out as I extracted a chunk of concrete from her infected ankle. We worked side by side with young paramedical volunteers. Wound after wound was cleansed, debrided, and dressed. Crushed and fractured limbs were assessed by palpation and functional status. Those fractured limbs that were ambulatory were treated with Ace wraps, and those that were not were reduced as close to an anatomic position as possible and splinted; the fractures were more than a week old, and Hopital General was only dealing with open devastating wounds and fractures.

A woman presented with an upper extremity crush injury. I am certain that she must have had compartment syndrome early on, but her limb and life were saved because the skin and tissues of her forearm split open. I amputated 3 digits and widely debrided necrotic tissue from her hand. As I operated, in a church courtyard, surrounded by curious children and an anxious sister, doing a case that in the United States would have been done under general anesthesia, she laid still and stoic without even a whimper. After the wound was dressed and a sling was applied, she thanked us effusively for a handful of ibuprofen, the first pain medicine she had received after 9 days of horrible pain. She returned to our host clinic for follow-up. The stumps were healing nicely, and the swelling in her hand was markedly reduced. Unfortunately, en route to the clinic she was caught in a motorcycle accident and sustained deep abrasions to her legs. We treated those wounds as well.

There were many dehydrated babies. Most of them were treated with oral rehydration and a few with IV rehydration. One baby was so badly dehydrated that we could not obtain IV access and had to revert to an old technique called hypodermoclysis, a subcutaneous infusion of fluids.

Two desperate parents brought their only surviving daughter to the *Klinik*; they had seen the crushing death of her 2 siblings. The girl was hyperventilating and had not slept since the event, so had the parents. We administered diphenhydramine for sedation and worked to calm her. We counseled her parents and taught the whole family breathing and relaxation exercises.

At our first Solino *Klinik*, a grandmother invited us into her sparse bedsheet tent to proudly show off her daughter's newborn infant. On our last day, I saw the grandmother gently plaiting her daughter's hair, and I inquired about the baby, *"Tibebe a mouri…"* The young mother, too dehydrated and malnourished, was unable to breast-feed. I did not know enough *Kreyòl* to properly give my condolences, but I sat for a few moments and shared their silence.

THREE MONTHS POSTEARTHQUAKE

A team of 6 members returned to Christ Roi in April 2010. It was a joyous reunion for returning team members, staff, and neighborhood acquaintances. HSJ was again our base. The building was being demolished by hand; men were working with pickaxes, crowbars, and sledgehammers. A temporary clinic with 2 examination rooms and a pharmacy was functioning 3 days a week on-site, and half-day school sessions, AM and PM, were being held, with all children receiving a hot lunch. A dormitory constructed of corrugated aluminum, with twin beds and fans, was now our home; flush toilets (with a bucket) and a shower (bucket bath) stall our amenities.

On this visit, we primarily assisted the Haitian primary care physicians and pediatricians in the HSJ clinic and also held clinics on their days off. We held one *Klinik Mobil* at a tent city in Pegueyville, outside Pètionville, at the request of 2 Brooklyn aid workers who had discovered a band of orphaned boys dropped off and abandoned at the site. We treated their wounds and worms and also saw the many women and children who queued for treatment. Our presence was announced by *radio bouch* (word of mouth), and so a motorcyclist dropped off a man with a freshly broken femur. We made him as comfortable as possible by laying him in the shade, reducing his limb, and giving him ibuprofen. Our transport van had gone on other errands, so it was not available. Shortly thereafter, a van with missionaries arrived, and we asked them to take the man to the hospital, but "it was out of their way." The missionaries took all the orphans, except for a boy with an open cleft palate and extremity deformities because he would be too much trouble. Abandoned again, now without his "wolf pack" for protection and aid, the child will surely die. At the end of the day, once our van returned, we transported the injured man to the hospital. The preoperative and postoperative tents of the DMAT were gone, but a good number of aid workers and tents remained, and in a more organized fashion. We expedited the injured man and his wife through the admission process, but the facility was reluctant to provide treatment.

We saw more than 500 patients on this trip; only 12% had surgical complaints, three-quarters had wounds and abscesses, and the remainder had hernias, congenital anomalies, and tumors. We treated the acute issues and referred the others to the Hopital; they probably will not be seen. The triune complaint of headache, stomach pain, and dizziness was pervasive. Most people were eating only 1 or 2 meager meals a day. New complaints of back pain echoed. At daytime, they were laboring to demolish or repair their homes, and at night, they were sleeping on the ground, some now with real tents. We could not provide food or better shelter, so we gave them over-the-counter pain relief and antacids; we added vitamins for everyone, young and old. Amazingly, despite malnutrition, dehydration, and gross contamination, wounds were healing well.

SIX MONTHS POSTEARTHQUAKE

We continue to learn from our experiences and have made more contacts. On this trip, we were able to acquire prescription medications for general medical and infective conditions. We also received many donations of a wider variety of over-the-counter medications. Although our treatments still remained largely symptomatic and palliative, we were able to advance to providing more focused medical care.

On a third trip to Haiti, we spent 1 day assisting in the HSJ clinic, which had now expanded to include a laboratory facility, an enlarged pharmacy, and a large sturdy tent with a triage area and 2 examination rooms. Because we had the perspective of time, the circumstances, and some familiarity with the staff, our role was not only to provide medical/surgical care but also to observe the *Klinik* system and make recommendations for improvements. We met with the visiting board members to discuss our suggestions. We also held *Klinik Mobil*, returning to the Acra neighborhood for 2 days, which was set up in a church just outside Cite Soleil (a notoriously dangerous slum) for 1 day. Clean water seemed to be readily available in P-a-P; however, the air was heavy with particulate matter, and there was an increase in respiratory and eye irritation complaints.

A mother brought her 2 desperately ill infants, both in acute respiratory distress with high fever. We initiated treatment with oral infant acetaminophen and antibiotics. We did not have a nebulizer, so we used metered dose inhaler treatments instead. Because of the severity of their illness, we transported them to Hopital General but were turned away because the ward was full of actively dying children. Our physician assistant dedicated hours to treating these children, with small doses of adult prednisone and oral rehydration. By the end of the day, they were much improved, but we had to leave; we have hope for the children but no knowledge of their outcome.

On this trip, we were invited to journey to a secluded mountain village, Fond Baptiste, perched high above the plain of Artibonite. Our trip took more than 4 hours, with half of the team balanced precariously atop supplies at the back of a 4-wheel drive pickup truck, vying with mules, goats, and pedestrians for the road. Health care was a distant memory to those people; however, the air was cool and clean but the water not as much. Extensive dental caries and worm infestations were common. We saw more elderly patients, most in surprisingly good health. But many untreated surgical conditions were observed in patients of all ages, especially hernias.

Our visit had been timed to coincide with the weekly market to maximize the number of patients we could see in a 2-day visit. By chance, after a walk through the market at the end of clinic hours, we came upon a woman with a large arm tumor, and she was sitting on her porch rocking in pain. On physical examination, the mass was 20 × 20 cm, firmly fixed to her upper humerus, and exquisitely tender on palpation. We gave her the only narcotics we had, from the private script of a team member, and invited her daughter to bring her to the clinic the next day. In the morning, she came for a formal visit. She had received a little relief from our medication but had slept a little, the first rest in quite awhile. We gave her all the remaining methocarbamol and ibuprofen from our pharmacy. We have been trying to make arrangements between our contacts in HSJ, Fond Baptiste, and a team of orthopedic physicians who provide service at Hospital Sacre Coeur in Milot near Cap Haïtien. Unfortunately, because of the plethora of intervening events in Haiti over the past 3 months, we have not been able to set up for her either a scheduled appointment or a travel to the distant site over harrowing roads; by the time we can make arrangements, it surely will be too late to be of benefit. If we are able to return to that location and she still lives, we will be certain to take some more potent medication especially for her.[23]

SUMMARY

Sometimes, our missions are like a series of throwing 1 starfish at a time into the vast ocean, an immeasurable task, but it is worth it all to the few starfish that are returned to their briny home. Despite their dire circumstances, our Haitian patients attend the Klinik looking their best, shoes polished, little girls' hair neatly braided, and young boys spiffed and polished. They are polite, enormously grateful for the simplest of examinations, and pleasantly surprised by our gift of vitamins to one and all. Perhaps, the greatest palliative care we provide is the assurance that there are still caring individuals in the world and the hope for a better tomorrow.

Palliative care is implemented in an individually designed fashion; disaster care is organized to provide the best for the most in austere circumstances. When these 2 elements struck head-on in a little known yet very locally accessible nation, with only a very basic infrastructure before the disaster, a challenging situation occurred. Preparation and planning on the part of those planning to deploy must include all aspects of emergency response, including palliative care. Yet, despite the proximity of Haiti, there had been little general education in the United States about the background of our sister nation; understanding the history and culture of a locale is essential to provide sensitive, appropriate care that will be accepted by the local population. Early wound and fracture intervention was key not only to help prevent progression to limb loss, sepsis, and death but also to increase mobility, a crucial necessity for homeless survivors who daily had to seek food and water.

When surgeons respond to a disaster situation, they will encounter suffering on an enormous scale. Although active triage and treatment are undertaken, in some instances, proper intervention is not an operation or primary disease control but to give comfort and restore hope. Palliative care can mean giving a man a stick to bite on while his leg is amputated, touching the shoulder of a mother whose child was buried under the collapse of the school building, or bringing a smile to the face of a child who has not smiled for 6 months.

EXTENDED CHALLENGES

As if all the past political and socioeconomic factors compounded by the tragic earthquake are not enough for the Haitian people to bear, hurricane force winds and rain, a cholera epidemic, and incendiary violence caused by an uncertain presidential election may further test Haiti's health care availability and function, as well as the ability for foreign nongovernmental organizations to safely be able to continue to gain access to the country and give ongoing care. For most Haitians, the experience of daily living is an exercise in palliative care. But they persevere saying, "beyond mountains there are more mountains," a common Haitian proverb that the natives live by—despite all the challenges they have had to overcome, there are yet more challenges to come, and still, they hope for a better future.

ACKNOWLEDGMENTS

The author wishes to acknowledge all the care providers who responded to Haiti in the hour of need and those who continue to respond. To give full credit to all the team members and volunteers who worked side by side with the author, please see the Men Anpil Web site (www.men-anpil.org).[24]

REFERENCES

1. WHO definition of palliative care. Available at: http://www.who.int/cancer/palliative/definition/en/. World Health Organization; 2010. Accessed December 19, 2010.
2. The White House. Homeland Security Presidential Directives/HSPD-21. Definition of catastrophic health event (i.e. mass casualty event). October 18, 2007. Available at: http://ncdmph.usuhs.edu/documents/hspd-21.pdf. Accessed December 19, 2010.
3. Briggs SM. The role of civilian surgical teams in response to international disasters. Bull Am Coll Surg 2010;95(1):13–7.
4. Smith P. 34. Blood dazzler. Minneapolis (MN): Coffee House Press; 2008.
5. Bogucki S, Jubanyik K. Triage, rationing and palliative care in disaster planning. Biosecur Bioterror 2009;7(2):221–4.
6. Elliot M. Haiti's agony. TIME Special Report: Haiti's tragedy. January 25, 2010: 30–6.
7. Clinton B. What Haiti needs. TIME Special Report: Haiti's tragedy. January 25, 2010: 37.
8. WHO/PAHO. Culture and mental health in Haiti: a literature review. Geneva (Switzerland): WHO; 2010.

9. World Statistics Pocketbook/United Nations Statistics Division. Last update in UN data: 14 May 2010. Available at: http://data.un.org/CountryProfile.aspx?crName= Haiti. (GNI data). Accessed January 7, 2011.

10. Central Intelligence Agency. The world factbook. (The on-line factbook is updated weekly) (poverty data). Available at: https://www.cia.gov/library/publications/the-world-factbook/geos/ha.html#top. Accessed December 19, 2010.

11. Responding to the Emergency at L'Hôpital Université d'État d'Haïti: a first step in rebuilding Haiti's public health care system. In: Proceedings of Friends of L'Hôpital Université d'État d'Haïti in conjunction with Partners in Health. March 31, 2010.

12. Ramnarace C. The forgotten victims: Haiti's elderly. AARP Bulletin. Available at: http://www.cynthiaramnarace.com/yahoo_site_admin/assets/docs/Help_for_Haiti_Earthquakes_0610.192115005.pdf. Accessed February 13, 2011.

13. de Montesquiou A. Elderly at Haiti hospice going without aid, waiting to die. Available at: http://www.huffingtonpost.com/2010/001/17/elderly-at-hospice_n_426324.html?view=screen. Accessed January 17, 2010.

14. Partners in health earthquake response. Available at: www.standwithhaiti.org. Accessed December 19, 2010.

15. Schneidman DS. Surgeons respond to the needs of a broken nation. Bull Am Coll Surg 2010;95(6):6–9, 12–20.

16. Etienne M, Powell C, Faux B. Disaster relief in Haiti: a perspective from the neurologists on the USNS COMFORT. 2010. Available at: www.thelancet.com/neurology. Accessed December 19, 2010.

17. Eastman AB. Haiti impressions. Bull Am Coll Surg 2010;95(6):9–11.

18. Ben-Achour S. Casualties and limits confront Navy Hospital Ship. Shots – NPR's Health Blog. Available at: http://www.npr.org/blogs/health/2010/01/casualties_and_limits_strike_h.html. Accessed January 24, 2010.

19. Kilgore C. Work in Haiti leaves mark on volunteers. American College of Surgeons. Surgery News March 2010;6(3):1, 4.

20. SCCM members provide relief to disaster victims. Critical Connections. SCCM 2010;9(2):1–117.

21. Critical care at a critical time. Critical Connections. SCCM 2010;9(2):8–9.

22. Oelkers N. Blog from the field: Haiti Feb 6-Feb 19. Operation Smile blog. Available at: http://www.operationsmile.org/haiti/haiti-week-2.html. Accessed February 14, 2010.

23. Hospice Saint Joseph. Available at: www.hospicesaintjoseph.org. Accessed December 19, 2010.

24. Author's Medical Mission Web site. Men Anpil (Many Hands). Available at: www.men-anpil.org. Accessed December 19, 2010.

Index

Note: Page numbers of article titles are in **boldface** type.

Surg Clin N Am 91 (2011) 459–465
doi:10.1016/S0039-6109(11)00025-9
0039-6109/11/$ – see front matter © 2011 Elsevier Inc. All rights reserved.

surgical.theclinics.com

Moving?

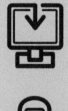

Moving?

Printed and bound by CPI Group (UK) Ltd, Croydon, CR0 4YY

03/10/2024

01040458-0020